HEALTHY SEX EDUCATION IN YOUR SCHOOLS

HEALTHY SEX EDUCATION IN YOUR SCHOOLS

A PARENTS' HANDBOOK

ANNE NEWMAN ▪ DINAH RICHARD

Focus on the Family Publishing
Pomona, CA 91799

First printing, 1990
Printed in the United States of America

Anne Newman and Dinah Richard
Healthy Sex Education in Your Schools: A Parents' Handbook
Summary: A manual for parents on working with public school personnel to implement abstinence education in classroom treatments of sex and family life instruction.

ISBN 0-929608-85-2

DEDICATED TO

Our children and their future children,
and all children.

ABOUT THE AUTHORS

Anne Newman is a wife, mother of two teenage boys and full-time homemaker. When Anne's boys were in middle school, she began to be concerned about some of the materials being used for their instruction. In 1986, in response to a specific novel which was being used in a class, Anne and some other parents were successful in having the book removed from the classroom. Next they worked with the school board to develop guidelines for supplemental reading assignments. Growing out of this effort, they formed a chapter of Citizens for Excellence in Education.

In the fall of 1988, Anne was instrumental in the school board's decision to adopt a policy that abstinence education be the standard taught in sex education. Through her work as president of the local chapter of Citizens for Excellence in Education (CEE), Anne has learned how to work effectively within the schools and the community. As a result, she has become a respected resource person in the Southwest. Anne and her husband John reside in San Antonio.

Dinah Richard is a wife, mother of four young children, and a full-time homemaker. Dinah holds a Ph.D. in speech communication and taught at the university level before resigning her position in order to stay home and raise her family.

Along with her family responsibilities, Dinah served as the volunteer director of a pro-life speaker's bureau. In 1985 she developed a strategy to reach public schools with information about the value of human life, the benefits of abstaining from premarital sex and the consequences of adolescent sex and abortion.

School officials began to request an increasing number of presentations about adolescent abstinence. Teachers, school nurses and counselors asked Dinah for information about the comparative success of abstinence education and contraceptive education. Motivated by this widespread interest, Dinah began to intensively research the subject. This effort culminated in the publication by Focus on the Family of

Has Sex Education Failed Our Teenagers? A Research Report. Dinah and her husband Conrad reside in San Antonio.

Dinah and Anne became acquainted in 1986 when they were both "novices" on the subject of sex education. Since then they have become good friends, attend the same church, and work together on special projects such as this handbook for parents.

CONTENTS

PREFACE xiii

ACKNOWLEDGMENTS xv

INTRODUCTION xvii

COUNT THE COST xxi

OVERVIEW xxv

I. GET ORGANIZED 1
A. Establish a Local Chapter of a National Organization
B. Establish a New Organization, Group, Council, or Committee
C. Organize a Coalition of Already-Existing Groups

II. GATHER INFORMATION 5
A. Become Informed About the General Issues of Sex Education
B. Become Informed About the Teenage Sexuality Crisis in Your Community
C. Become Informed About the Education at the State Level
D. Become Informed About Your Local School District
E. Find Out Where Abstinence Education Is Offered Elsewhere
F. Find Out About Textbooks

III. EVALUATE YOUR SCHOOL DISTRICT'S SEX EDUCATION PROGRAM 15
A. Arrange to Examine the Sex Education Materials
B. Write a Critique of the District's Sex Education Program
C. Criteria for Evaluating Your School's Sex Education Program

IV. DECIDE WHAT NEEDS TO BE DONE IN THE SCHOOLS 31
A. Propose a Good Policy for the School District
B. Propose Good Guidelines for the School District
C. Propose a Good Protocol for the District

V. MAKE YOUR CASE IN WRITING 35
A. Put Together a Case
B. Put Together a Promotional Packet

VI. CONTACT THE SCHOOL'S KEY DECISION-MAKERS 37
A. Set Up Appointments
B. Go to the Meeting
C. Persuade People to Read the Sex Education Report

VII. RECRUIT COMMUNITY SUPPORT FOR YOUR PROPOSAL 41
A. People to Approach
B. How to Approach Groups and Individuals
C. Channel Public Opinion Back to Key Decision-Makers
D. Keep the Public Updated on Your Progress

VIII. WORK WITH THE MEDIA 45
A. Tips for Media Contacts
B. Letters to the Editor
C. Press Releases
D. Holding a Press Conference
E. Television
F. Talking to Reporters
G. Radio Interviews
H. News Programs
I. Radio Talk Shows
J. Other Ways to Work With the Media

IX. SHARPEN YOUR STRATEGY 53
A. Dealing With Opposition
B. Maintain Contact With Key Decision-Makers
C. Consider Timing of School Board Elections

X. GO BEFORE THE BOARD 55
A. Who Serves on the Board?
B. The School Board's Role
C. The Importance of Citizen Interaction With the School Board
D. How to Identify Board Members' Positions on the Issues
E. Develop a Board Member Or Candidate Survey
F. The Voting Patterns of the Board
G. Influencing the School Board
H. Bring the Issue Before a Board Meeting
I. Addressing the School Board

XI. IF YOU WIN, FOLLOW THROUGH 63
A. Reinforcing the Policy
B. Monitoring Policy Implementation
C. Sex Education Committee
D. Handling Complaints and Problem Areas
E. A Final Area of Concern: Your State

XII. IF YOU LOSE, THEN WHAT? 67
A. Work to Elect Board Members Who Represent Your Views
B. Keep Up Public Pressure
C. Counter Negative Teaching
D. Excuse Your Child From an Objectionable Program
E. Set Up a Lending Library and Speakers Bureau
F. Hold Community Based Abstinence Programs
G. Hold Teacher Training Conferences

XIII. SCHOOL BOARD ELECTIONS 71
A. Organize Candidate Selection Committee
B. Guidelines for Selection of Candidates
C. Develop and Use a Candidate Screening Survey
D. Host a "Meet the Candidates Night"
E. Suggestions to Help Elect Candidates

XIV. CONCLUSION 75

APPENDICES 77
A. Set Up a Prayer Network
B. Differing Views: What People Think of Each Other
C. Tips for Gathering Information by Phone
D. The Teenage Sexuality Crisis in the Community
E. Programs for Teens in the Community
F. The State's Education Structure
G. State Laws About Sex Education
H. Locating Information in the District
I. School District Information
J. The School's Sex Education Program
K. Abstinence Programs Elsewhere in Your Region
L. Evaluating Your School's Sex Education Program
M. Giving a Talk Before an Audience
N. Useful Verses to Review Before Speaking
O. Outline of a Sample Talk
P. Common Arguments and How to Answer Them
Q. Complaint Inquiry
R. Specific Helps for Parents and Guiding Principles
S. Sample Petition
T. Sample Letters to the Editor
U. Sample Press Releases
V. Sample School Board Candidate Screening Forms
W. Publishers of Abstinence Education Materials
X. Periodicals that Cover Education Issues
Y. National Organizations that Have Local Chapters
Z. Glossary of Terms
AA. Books to Guide Parents
BB. Audiovisual Resources for Adults on Teenage Sexuality
CC. Books for Teens
DD. Tapes for Teens
EE. Books to Help Parents Teach Children
FF. Tapes to Help Parents Teach Children
GG. Pamphlets to Help Parents Teach Children

PREFACE

"Help me! Planned Parenthood is coming to our school. What should I do?"

"I'm shocked at what my daughter showed me in her biology text. Can I do anything to influence what the school is teaching?"

"I've been appointed to our school's sex education committee. How can I convince the school to adopt abstinence education, not contraceptive education?"

"I want to play an active role in the schools regarding sex education. Where do I start?"

These are typical problems that Christian parents face today. If you are in a similar circumstance, you are not alone. Sex education is taught in most schools across the country, but often, it is taught from the wrong approach. Painful and costly experience has shown that sex education which is separated from clear moral and ethical values is not effective. Such instruction has actually been shown to worsen the problems of teen pregnancy and sexually transmitted diseases (STDs).

Now that quality education materials which advocate sexual abstinence are available, schools can provide an approach that works. Unfortunately, parents are sometimes the only ones who take the initiative to influence the schools toward a sound policy in handling sex education. With the many responsibilities that parents already have, the task of trying to change a school's approach can seem overwhelming. Yet when practical steps are presented to them, ordinary parents have taken on this vital issue with a high degree of success.

This parents' manual was developed to help parents become involved in encouraging their public schools to implement an effective abstinence education program. Also available from Focus on the Family Publishing are:

- *Has Sex Education Failed Our Teenagers? A Research Report.* This volume was written primarily for public school officials with application to other public policy-makers. It is a very effective tool for you to place in the hands of key policy-makers. It provides extensive evidence from educational research which shows conclusively that contraceptive education is a failed strategy while abstinence education has proven effective.
- *Family Values and Sex Education.* Because pre-adolescents are at increasingly high risk from the problems which result from teenage sexual activity, this curriculum is targeted at middle school students. F.V.S.E. is the result of a major cooperative effort among national leaders in quality education. It sensitively and

creatively presents a clear message of the benefits of abstinence for all young people.

The sex education report and the *F.V.S.E.* curriculum are designed for use in any school, public or private. This Parents' Handbook is written from a Christian perspective to help you plan and carry out an effective approach to school personnel.

Although this Handbook concentrates on sex education in the schools, the principles and procedure are general enough so that they can be applied to other educational issues which concern you.

One of the authors of the manual, along with a few other concerned parents, began working to improve their school district's sex education. They took a few steps at a time. Since they did not have a handbook such as this, they had to learn along the way. Their experiences contributed many of the tips contained in these pages, making sure you have all the information you might need and the procedures you might need to pursue.

When Time is Limited
...Take the Basic Steps!

While the amount of information and suggested action in this manual may seem overwhelming, do not be alarmed. It is not necessary to do everything listed in the manual to achieve success. A few steps taken by a few committed parents can have a positive impact.

Each section of this handbook is introduced with a few "Basic Steps"—actions which are crucial to the success of your efforts. You will not need to do everything this handbook suggests, but if you truly want to make a difference, thoughtfully consider all the "Basic Steps."

ACKNOWLEDGMENTS

We thank God for the help and guidance He has provided through these people:

The board members of our local Citizens for Excellence in Education (CEE) chapter who gave their time, prayers and encouragement as we learned and grew together;

Ron Johnson for making the sacrifice and commitment to run for school board two consecutive years to achieve victory; and for helping to make an abstinence sex education policy in our district possible.

Our husbands (John and Conrad) for their loving encouragement during this endeavor.

The many friends who helped and encouraged us.

Dinah would also like to express her appreciation to her parents, Guy and Doris Daniel, for taking care of her four children while she worked on this manual.

Special thanks to the people who read and commented on our writing: Joyce Andreas, Dr. Tom and Laurie Fitch, Mike Hill, John Newman, Conrad Richard, and Susan Weddington who gave valuable advice regarding the media.

INTRODUCTION

It is important that we understand what has happened to our society and how we can have a part in the solution.

We must understand the times we are living in and discover what we should do.

Some 28 years ago an ordinary couple from Longview, Texas, Mel and Norma Gabler, discovered inaccuracies in their sons' textbooks. Mel told Norma that she had to go to Austin, the seat of the Texas State Board of Education and the Texas Education Agency. Norma asked, "What will I do when I get there?" Mel replied, "I don't know, but you've got to do something!"

Many parents feel the same uncertainty of what to do, and the same conviction that something must be done. Our common sense and our values tell us that something is wrong in the way sex education is being taught.

At first parents tend to assume that just pointing out the problem will be enough. "If I mention it to the teacher or bring it to the principal's attention, they'll fix it." Many parents soon learn that when they discuss moral standards and values, they are labelled "fundamentalists" and told that they cannot impose their morals on all the students. It's the old argument: "You can't legislate morality." Many Christian parents back away at this point, unsure of what to do.

As we look around us, we tend to see symptoms of deeper, underlying problems. Our attention is caught by the specter of child abuse, by the AIDS epidemic, by drug addiction, by violent crime, by the high rate of teenage pregnancy.

Our nation has turned its back on God, and we are reaping the results in a host of societal problems. As He has done over the centuries, God is calling us back to himself. "If my people, who are called by my name, will humble themselves and pray and seek my face and turn from their wicked ways, then will I hear from heaven and will forgive their sin and will heal their land." 2 Chronicles 7:14

Most of us remember Jesus' words: "You are the salt of the earth. But if the salt loses its saltiness, how can it be made salty again?" How many can recall the next sentence? "It is no longer good for anything, except to be thrown out and trampled by men." Matthew 5:13. Our Christian values have been trampled. Christians have allowed the "salt" to lose its flavor. When used properly, salt is a preservative.

Christians, when we choose, can help preserve society.

Nehemiah found himself in a situation which parallels ours. The wall of Jerusalem was in ruins, leaving the city unprotected. Nehemiah "wept and mourned" because of the "great distress and reproach" of Jerusalem in such a sad state. Nehemiah spent days praying and fasting about Jerusalem. After four months, he realized he had a part in the answer to his prayer, and he called his countrymen to help rebuild the walls.

The spectacle of Jerusalem with its broken walls, rubble, and burned gates provides a graphic picture of what has happened to our society. Our families' first line of defense—morality, authority, integrity, and decency based on Biblical principles—has been torn down. In the wall of Jerusalem were many gates with different purposes. One gate, the Refuse Gate, was used to remove garbage to the Valley Hinnom to be burned. Like Jerusalem, our system of removing garbage from our society has broken down. The "trash" of our society—violence, pornography, corruption, drugs, and immorality on TV, in music, literature, etc.—is building up and the stench is destroying our society.

For example, the Supreme Court's 1962 decision against prayer in school was a benchmark event. Since that time we have seen many evidences of drastic decline in the life of our nation. David Barton in his book, *America: To Pray or Not to Pray,* documents many of the negative trends of the intervening years. Barton shows the drop in SAT scores, the rise in sexually transmitted disease, unwed teen pregnancy, suicide, crime rates, divorce rates, child abuse reports, and illegal drug use.[1] It presents a chilling picture of a nation which does not honor God.

> *"For although they knew God, they neither glorified him as God nor gave thanks to him; but their thinking became futile, and their foolish hearts were darkened. Although they claimed to be wise, they became fools. . . . Therefore God gave them over in the sinful desires of their hearts to sexual impurity for the degrading of their bodies with one another."* Romans 1:21-24.

YOUR RESPONSIBILITY

> *"These commandments that I give you today are to be upon your hearts. Impress them on your children. Talk about them when you sit at home and when you walk along the road, when you lie down and when you get up."* Deuteronomy 6:6,7

After Norma Gabler cited many errors and contradictions in several economic textbooks at a State Board of Education hearing, one board member asked, "What are your qualifications? Why should we listen to anything you have to say?" Norma replied, "Sir, I am a mother of three sons. I pay taxes from which these books are purchased. I vote to elect the member of this Board from my district. Can you think of three better reasons?"[3]

"You have the right to demand for your children the best our schools and colleges can provide. Your vigilance and your refusal to be satisfied with less than the best are the imperative first step." *A Nation at Risk*[2]

Many parents let themselves believe that the professionals know more than parents. As a result the role of educating our children has often been surrendered to the professionals. A closer scrutiny of our children's education is needed, especially since public schools have been thrust into the role of dealing with the social ills of society.

Schools have taken on the responsibility of sex education, often because of the common rationale, "the parents aren't doing it." Some parents have asked the schools to do it, while others, burdened with their own troubles, have been relieved that the schools are doing it. Sadly, the evidence continues to mount that the approach most schools have taken has proven ineffective at best.

If we are distressed about the problems we see around us, we must, like Nehemiah, petition God as well as see our part in rebuilding the broken walls. As parents we must accept the God-given responsibility of our children's moral and ethical education. We must be willing to ask questions, look for answers, challenge ineffective and harmful programs, and support efforts which are effective. We must devote our time and effort to this task.

> As parents we have the primary, inalienable right to educate our children according to our religious, moral and cultural values. We delegate, but do not abdicate, that right to schools and teachers. We are accountable to God for our children. This parental responsibility requires that we demand excellence in all areas of education.
>
> We entrust teachers with the awesome responsibility of teaching future generations of Americans. They need and deserve our support and cooperation.
>
> Schools must respect parental rights and actively seek to encourage parental involvement in every area of education. School boards, administrators, and teachers are accountable to the taxpayers and parents who support them and entrust their children to them. (Adapted from Citizens for Excellence in Education Manual)

Footnotes

[1] *America: To Pray or Not to Pray,* David Barton, Specialty Research Associates, Inc., P.O. Box 397, Aledo, TX

[2] *A Nation At Risk: The Imperative for Educational Reform,* a Report to the Nation and the Secretary of Education Department of Education by the National Commission on Excellence in Education, April 1983.

[3] *What Are They Teaching Our Children?* Mel and Norma Gabler.

COUNT THE COST

"Suppose one of you wants to build a tower. Will he not first sit down and estimate the cost to see if he has enough money to complete it?"

Luke 14:28

Before taking on a challenge, first consider what it will involve:

COMMITMENT

"Commit to the Lord whatever you do,
and your plans will succeed." Proverbs 16:3

Once you have sought the Lord's guidance, it is essential to make a commitment to work toward accomplishing His purposes. Bringing about positive changes in the public schools will take time and effort. It will probably require an investment of time and energy and may be a long-term project. Are you willing to commit yourself to this effort?

How Will This Affect Your Family?

How will your children handle it if their friends tease them by calling their parents "moral" as if "moral" is a dirty word? How will they handle it if teachers make disparaging comments? How will you handle it? Discussing what may happen can reduce problems later.

Can You Handle Defeat?

Sometimes we expect instant success because we are doing something good. We look for God to grant us victory every time. However, we fail to see His long term plan and greater purpose.

What you may see as a defeat can be setting the stage for a later victory. Through your struggles, you will grow stronger. You will meet and help others, and be helped by them. You will witness to those you might prefer to avoid. You will realize your weaknesses and strengths. You will learn more about God than you know now. Are you willing to face opposition and possibly be humbled through defeat?

Can You Stand Alone?

"I am the only one left, and now they are trying to kill me too." 1 Kings 19:14

There may be times that you will feel like you are the only one who cares about this issue. You will feel how Elijah felt, and how Nehemiah must have felt when some people refused to join in rebuilding the wall (Nehemiah 3:5). Those you expect to be supportive may disappoint you. A favorite Sunday school teacher once said, "Right is right, even if nobody is doing it. Wrong is wrong, even if everybody is doing it." This is still a good principle to follow.

Can You Handle Ridicule?

Nehemiah and his "wall-builders" were mocked and called feeble (Nehemiah 4:1,2).

Mel and Norma Gabler have been ridiculed and maligned by textbook publishers, educators and the media. They have been labelled every imaginable name, including "ignorant, fear-mongering, right-wing fruitloops." Although the Gablers have never censored one book, they have been accused of "censoring textbooks." They and their professional staff carefully examine textbooks considered for adoption in Texas. They testify at textbook hearings concerning inaccuracies, distortions and biases. They show that traditional American values, such as the work ethic, free enterprise and the importance of the family as the basic social unit have been "censored" from textbooks.

Parents who oppose the existing system have been referred to as "fundamentalists," "extremists," "radical," "smother-mother," "not living in a real world," "head buried in the sand" and "censors." They have been accused of quenching academic freedom, wanting to take education back to the Dark Ages and depriving children of true learning.

SACRIFICE

"The strength of the laborers is giving out. . ." Nehemiah 4:10

Nehemiah's building work was attacked by conspiracy (Nehemiah 4:7-23), by extortion (5:1-19), by compromise (6:1-4), by slander (6:5-9), and by treachery (6:10-14).

It has been said that anything worth doing is worth doing right, and there is always a cost involved in any worthwhile endeavor. Expect this effort to cost you time, effort and money. Are you willing to make sacrifices of these limited resources? Is your family willing to make sacrifices?

A WORD OF ENCOURAGEMENT

"I can do everything through him who gives me strength."
Philippians 4:13

Counting the cost is necessary to be prepared for what is ahead. Rather than being an exercise in discouragement, counting the cost helps you sense your need for God's help. As you sense that need, you become increasingly aware of God's strength at work through your weakness.

Nehemiah was aware of "the gracious hand of my God upon me" (Nehemiah 2:18). He was thus able to challenge his people: "Don't be afraid of them. Remember the Lord, who is great and awesome, and fight for your brothers, your sons and your daughters, your wives and your homes" (Nehemiah 4:14). As a result, the work was accomplished in 52 days! When the enemies heard of it, they "lost their self-confidence, because they realized that this work had been done with the help of our God" (Nehemiah 6:16).

THE HIGH COST OF NON-INVOLVEMENT

Finally, we would not be completely honest with you if we did not remind you of the cost of not getting involved. The stakes are very high. By not speaking up, we risk our children and our neighbors' children. We risk immense continuing damage to our society by ill-informed, maladjusted men and women of tomorrow. We risk the anguish of failing to do what our loving, heavenly Father desires. And we give up the joy and reward God has planned for those who are faithful!

OVERVIEW

SEE THE TOTAL PROCESS

Let's get a broad picture of what a person or group would need to do in order to influence the school system. The following chart previews the steps aimed at the adoption of a policy that upholds abstinence in all sex education efforts. We have devoted a complete chapter to each step in this process.

1. GET ORGANIZED WITH OTHERS
2. GATHER INFORMATION *
3. EVALUATE THE SCHOOL'S PROGRAM *
4. DECIDE WHAT NEEDS TO BE DONE IN THE SCHOOLS
5. PREPARE YOUR CASE
6. ESTABLISH INITIAL CONTACT WITH THE SCHOOL'S KEY DECISION-MAKERS *
7. RECRUIT COMMUNITY SUPPORT
8. WORK WITH THE MEDIA
9. SHARPEN YOUR STRATEGY
10. GO BEFORE THE BOARD
11. IF YOU WIN, FOLLOW THROUGH
12. IF YOU LOSE, THEN WHAT?
13. SCHOOL BOARD ELECTIONS

Don't be overwhelmed by the length of this manual! Look first at the suggested "Basic Steps" at the front of each chapter, then proceed further into that section if that topic addresses your circumstances.

***NOTE:** The topics marked with an asterisk (*) are the ones on which to focus if you have limited time or objectives. See "But I'm All Alone and I Have Only One Week" on the next page.

We have also added worksheets, resources and practical helps in the appendices. We've included more than enough information to help you through each part of your task. We have tried to record the principles and techniques that we have used in our own interaction with schools over the past few years.

"BUT I'M ALL ALONE AND I HAVE ONLY ONE WEEK"

One of the major recommendations of this handbook is that you join forces with other parents, school personnel and community leaders who share your concern. However, you might not have time to get other parents organized with you and there may be no existing organizations in your community ready to get involved. Thus you find that you must stand alone. If you are under such a time constraint, you can still take effective action on short notice. Regardless of the reason that you are standing alone, don't become discouraged. Across the nation, there are many ordinary parents who have successfully stood alone in approaching the schools and the community. Usually, such people report that they later found out that there were many parents who admired what they were doing but didn't have the courage to speak up. Ultimately, we will all have to stand alone one day—before our maker—and He will ask us what we did, not what others did.

The Basic Steps

We have included special help in this manual for the parents who have only a short amount of time in which to accomplish a goal. If your immediate target is to extinguish a fire, such as removing an objectionable film, speaker, or book, and you have only a few days in which to do so, follow the advice in the "Basic Steps" section at the front of each chapter.

2. Gather Information
A. Become Informed About the General Issues of Sex Education
B. Become Informed About the State Level of Education
C. Become Informed About Your Local School District

3. Evaluate Your School's Sex Education Program
A. Arrange to See the Materials
B. Prepare a Written Critique

6. Establish Initial Contact With the School's Key Decision-Makers
A. Set Up Appointments
B. Go to the Meeting
C. Persuade People to Read the Sex Education Report

If you work through the above steps and you still have not been able to get the school to remove the objectionable materials, then proceed to the next step:

7. Recruit Community Support
If the school still does not remove the objectionable materials, then proceed to the next step.

continued on next page

The Basic Steps *continued*

10. Go Before the Board

If you achieve your immediate goal at any step in the process, be aware that you have probably won only a temporary victory. Read the preliminary paragraphs in "4. Decide What Needs to Be Done in the Schools." It points out that a favorable decision is good for the moment, but that a solid policy needs to be adopted to keep similar problems from occurring again. For that reason, whether or not you achieve your immediate short-range goal, you should eventually consider following through with a long-range plan, as described in the rest of Chapter 4.

Also review the Specific Helps for Parents and the Guiding Principles in Appendix R.

1
GET ORGANIZED

"Make plans by seeking advice;
if you wage war, obtain guidance."

Proverbs 20:18

BASIC STEPS:

If you are under time constraints and do not have the opportunity to set up an organization, you can still—

1. Get together with several other concerned parents in order to work together to accomplish your goal.
2. Ask several friends to pray for your efforts.
3. Contact a national organization and inform them of what you are doing. They may know people in your area who would assist you.

A desire to bring about positive changes in the schools may begin in the heart of one person, but there is a need for an organized effort. One or two parents can be easily ignored; it is more difficult to ignore an organized effort. An organized group can issue press releases, raise funds, and have a name with which those in the community can identify. Some options are:

A. ESTABLISH A LOCAL CHAPTER OF A NATIONAL ORGANIZATION

Establishing a local chapter of an organization allows you to build upon the established credibility and reputation of the national organization. Non-profit status has already been established which in some states allows you to purchase materials or printing tax-free. A bulk mail permit, which allows you to mail 200 pieces or more at special rates, can be more easily obtained. A national organization can provide information and resources.

Ask about officer and membership requirements, and how chapters operate in relationship to the national organization. For example, does every project and press release need approval from the national office? (See Appendix Y for addresses of national organizations.)

B. ESTABLISH A NEW ORGANIZATION, GROUP, COUNCIL, OR COMMITTEE

A group can be formed for the specific purpose of getting a particular policy passed or a program adopted. A group or organization can begin with five or six people who will agree to take a leadership position on the board of directors. The group can decide what positions need to be filled (Director, Assistant Director, Activity Director, Secretary, Treasurer, Research Director, etc.). More than one secretary may be needed. You can add positions or committees as necessary. Qualifications for board members and new board members should be determined by the board only. Board members should have a reputation for integrity, reliability and hard work.

Your essential purpose should be stated in writing and bylaws should be developed as guidelines for how you will operate. For example, is the organization to be a Christian one?

In choosing the name, consider what the initials might spell. The name should be generic enough to have wide appeal, but specific enough to identify the purpose. A name with a positive message is best when you are promoting a policy or program, i.e., "Citizens for" is better than "Citizens Against." The name should encourage the widest participation. "Citizens" would include taxpayers, grandparents, and civic leaders. "Parents" would exclude these.

C. ORGANIZE A COALITION OF ALREADY-EXISTING GROUPS

Forming a coalition of organizations, groups, and churches who share your goals can enhance credibility, divide the work load and reach more people. This could be done by asking each organization to promote the effort and supply one or two persons to work directly on the project as well as being a liaison to the organization.

Groups can work together behind the scenes to spread information, and they can develop a joint public effort. A joint press conference can be held to publicize the effort.

Care should be taken in selecting participants of a coalition. It is not necessary to be in agreement on all the issues, but alliances should be carefully considered. Also, if all the groups in the coalition are conservative Christian groups, then the coalition can be labelled the "religious right." It is helpful to include civic groups to provide a balance, as long as they share your same objectives.

TIPS FOR ORGANIZING A GROUP:

1. **Letterhead** for the group can be developed on a computer and copies can be made for just a few cents each. You may know friends who cannot commit to being on the board of directors, but will serve as consultants. Their names can be listed in the margin of the letterhead after the names of board members.

2. **A regular newsletter** is helpful in keeping your group informed and it can be sent to local pastors, leaders of the parent groups, and concerned citizens' organizations. Care should be taken in writing a newsletter. All information should be verified. Report some information as a person's opinion or statement, not as fact. A newsletter is generally most effective when it is published at regular intervals (i.e., the first of each month).

   Using an official sounding name such as "Education News" will allow you to send one of your "reporters" to seminars, meetings, school board conventions, teacher workshops, and other education events. Some events such as conventions will require a press badge which will be provided for you, but should be arranged for in advance. Other events will admit you when you identify yourself. It is best to call about the event in advance and ask if media will be allowed, if there is special seating, and if a "press pass" is needed.

3. **Set up a prayer network** within your organization. Refer to Appendix A for advice and a sample prayer request sheet.

4. **Review Specific Helps for Parents and Guiding Principles in Appendix R.**

Once organized, group members should set goals, plan strategy, and encourage others to join their efforts. Regular meetings should be held. Coalition participants can put information in their newsletters, make announcements at their meetings, communicate through phone chains, etc.

2

GATHER INFORMATION

"The heart of the discerning one acquires knowledge; the ears of the wise one seek it out."

Proverbs 18:15

Regardless of whether or not you are working with a group, you need to gather certain pieces of information before you try to influence the schools. If you are working with a group, delegate to several people the job of gathering the information you need at this stage. Assign each person a category listed below, send them on their way, and agree to meet together by a specific date.

BASIC STEPS:

If you are working alone or do not have time to gather all the information suggested in this chapter, don't abandon ship. Instead, gather the most pertinent information—

1. State laws about sex education;
2. The details of your school district's sex education program;
3. The names of school districts in your state where abstinence education is being offered.

A. BECOME INFORMED ABOUT THE GENERAL ISSUES OF SEX EDUCATION

Most parents realize that there are moral problems facing young people. However, they are often unaware about the ways in which family planning and sex education have contributed to this problem. Perhaps parents have had the opportunity to view some of the materials used in the schools, but they can't quite convey why they object to the program. For that reason, it is important for as many parents as possible to read through *Has Sex Education Failed Our Children? A Research Report,* also published by Focus on the Family.

1. Read *Has Sex Education Failed Our Teenagers? A Research Report.*

Become familiar with the arguments presented in the report. It will be your ammunition when working with the schools. While the report is intended to be given to school leaders, **do not give the report to school officials yet.** For now, you and other parents read it to help you become familiar with the topic and the key issues involved.

The sex education report is designed for school personnel such as teachers, nurses, principals, counselors, directors, superintendents, board members and other decision-makers. It also has application to health care workers, community leaders, clergy, legislators, and other people in the community who must make decisions regarding the selection of sex education programs and policies.

One of the underlying assumptions of the report is that most decision makers are more familiar with the wrong approaches to sex education—i.e., value-neutral education, values clarification, non-directive decision making, comprehensive sex education, contraceptive counseling, etc.. Decision makers need the evidence in this report which shows them why abstinence education is the more effective approach.

The sex education report has many advantages. It consolidates many studies drawn from various sources. A synthesis of studies becomes an advantage to school personnel because it relieves them from having to do extensive research, which would often be prohibitive due to their already overloaded schedule. You should point out this advantage when you hand the report to school personnel at the appropriate time.

Another advantage to the report is that it does not read like a novel. Instead, the reader can pick it up, flip through the report, and read any section. The report contains broad headings, subheadings, etc., for the sake of helping the reader understand the logical arrangement of materials, ideas, and arguments.

The report is written in neutral, non-inflammatory language. Though the report clearly defends abstinence education, the style of writing is non-emotional. This approach will help decision makers realize that abstinence education can be defended from a factual, rational perspective. Hopefully this will help to reduce any misconceptions that decision-makers will have about the advocates of abstinence education.

Likewise, the evidence cited in the report is taken from sources that educators deem to be credible. For example, a substantial portion of the information is drawn from major medical journals rather than publications (such as pro-life newsletters) that the reader would perceive to be biased. Also, when reviewing the failure of family planning, school-based clinics, and comprehensive sex education, the report deliberately cites information from pro-contraceptive publications. These citations show that even the research and statements by pro-contraceptive groups admit that their approaches are not effective.

The layout of the report is designed to make it inviting to read. The body of the report is broken up with frequent headings, charts, etc. to help move the reader through the text. The many tables help the reader quickly comprehend important statistical information.

Finally, the report lists resources that can be readily adopted into the classroom. Since schools have ready access to materials from the **wrong** approach, it is vital to bring to their attention the resources that follow the **right** approach.

As you and other parents read through the sex education report and become informed about the general issue of sex education, you are getting ready to knowledgeably pursue your goal of improving the sex education procedures in your school.

Appendix X
Periodicals That Cover Education Issues

Appendix AA
Books to Guide Parents

Appendix W
Publishers of Abstinence Education Materials

2. Keep Informed by Reading Other Resources.

To keep informed about educational issues, take out a subscription to one or more of the periodicals listed in Appendix X at the end of this handbook. Also, read some of the books listed in Appendix AA. In addition, ask to be placed on the mailing lists of publishers of abstinence materials, listed in Appendix W.

3. Keep Informed by Listening to Christian Radio Stations.

Christian radio programs can provide you with information about current issues. Some programs deal with national issues while others deal with problems in your locality. If your local stations are not adequately addressing these issues, write to them urging them to do so.

B. BECOME INFORMED ABOUT THE TEENAGE SEXUALITY CRISIS IN YOUR COMMUNITY

Besides becoming informed about the general issue of sex education, find out about the situation in your community. This information will prove helpful—

- when someone opposes you, saying, "But you are simply a parent. You don't understand the situation in our community."
- when you are trying to recruit support for your proposal, and people may claim that other agencies in the community are better equipped to handle the situation.
- as you begin to discuss the issue of sex education and seemingly credible people toss around statistics and references to various community organizations. In the presence of school decision makers, you might feel as though you are unable to defend your views because you don't know what the others are talking about.

The way to avoid these situations is to do some homework. By placing a few phone calls, you can get basic information that will help you better understand what is occurring in your community. If possible, delegate this step to someone who will share the information with those involved.

1. The Teenage Pregnancy Problem in Your Community

In order to determine the nature of the teenage sexuality crisis in your community, contact at least several of the following sources for information about teen pregnancy in your community:

State department of health
State department of human resources
State department of education
City or county health department
City or county department of human resources
Public and private child welfare agencies in your community
The director of health for your school district

The director of nursing for your school district
Family planning clinics in your community
Crisis pregnancy clinics in your community
Chapters of professional associations (for nurses, for physicians, for educators, for social workers)

Realize that the information you receive from these sources might be slanted toward approaches that you don't favor (i.e., abortion, contraceptives for minors without parental consent, etc.).

When contacting the agencies listed above, ask for information about:

the teenage population in your community,
the teenage pregnancies in your area,
teenage abortions,
teenage births,
school dropouts,
sexually transmitted diseases,
any other pertinent demographic data about teenagers in your community.

For your convenience, as you contact the above agencies, use the form in Appendix D at the end of this handbook. Some of the data that you obtain will not fit into the form, so adapt the form as needed. Be sure to make several photocopies of the blank form before you start your calls. Ask for any pamphlets and photocopies of all data. Always, make sure to cite the source of information (book, publisher, date, page number, author, etc.).

Review the advice in Appendix C on how to gather information by phone.

Appendix D
The Teenage Sexuality Crisis in the Community

Appendix C
Tips for Gathering Information by Phone

2. Sexuality Services for Teens in Your Community

In order to find out what information dissemination and services are available to teens in your community, make some more phone calls. Find out the extent of access teens in your community have to:

family planning services to teens,
abortions for teens,
counseling for pregnant teens,
homes for pregnant teens,
parenting classes for pregnant teens,
lending libraries that offer films about teenage sexuality and related topics,
groups that send speakers into the schools,
organizations that provide free literature about pregnancy and birth, etc.

Realize that some of the services and information available might oppose your values, so be sure to evaluate all organizations and their programs.

Here are a few of the sources to check to see if they offer sexuality information or services to teens:

public schools
private schools
universities
medical schools
hospitals
clinics
social service agencies
charities
pediatricians
obstetricians and gynecologists
family physicians
churches
para-church organizations
halfway houses
adoption agencies
counseling centers
pro-life groups
crisis pregnancy centers
civic organizations
youth clubs
prepared childbirth instructors

For each group, organization, or program, prepare a summary that lists: name of organization, contact person, address, phone, objective of the organization, affiliation, beliefs of the organization, description of the program or services that deal with teenage sexuality, whether the organization interacts with the public schools, its success in dealing with the teenage sexuality crisis, etc.

For convenience, use the form in Appendix E in order to fill in the information when placing phone calls. Be sure to make several photocopies of the blank form before you start your calls. These forms can be placed in your files once they are completed.

Review the advice in Appendix C on how to gather information by phone.

Appendix E
Programs for Teens in the Community

Appendix C
Tips for Gathering Information by Phone

C. BECOME INFORMED ABOUT EDUCATION AT THE STATE LEVEL

One parent asked the school teacher why students were being taught about contraception. The teacher replied, "Because it's required by state law." The parent backed off, assuming the teacher was correct. Later, the parent found out that no such law existed; there was simply a general mandate to teach human growth and reproduction. As it passed down through the chain of command, the law became misunderstood.

Therefore, before approaching school personnel, do some homework. Find out about the state's educational structure and the state laws about sex education. When someone claims the law requires a specific procedure, ask to see a copy of the law or policy that requires it.

Don't let this step become discouraging or overwhelming. Sometimes just making a few phone calls is all you have to do. Even though most of your calls will be placed to bureaucracies, don't let their "run-around" treatment frighten or discourage you. Most of the information you need probably can be obtained by calling your state education agency, which is usually in the capital. You may be able to get the information from your local district.

As you gather information, you may find someone who is willing to help you. An "insider" is invaluable in understanding the "ins and outs" of the system.

1. The Educational Code

Most states have an education code which can be reviewed at the school district office, local library, or purchased from the state. Some states have "essential elements" which can be very vague, and can be used as an excuse to teach such things as contraceptive education. Therefore, it is vital for you to obtain the exact wording of the state law. For convenience, use the form in Appendix G to learn the questions to ask about the state laws concerning sex education.

Appendix G
State Laws About
Sex Education

2. The Educational Structure

It is also important to find out about your state's educational structure. Finding out about the hierarchy and governing bodies will help you see how your local school district fits into the total picture. For your convenience, use the form in Appendix F when making your calls.

Appendix F
The State's
Education Structure

3. The Penal Code

You might also want to find out about your state penal code regarding sodomy, lawful marriage, deviant behavior, sexual intercourse among minors, parental consent, pornography, and homosexual issues. For example, is lawful marriage a marriage between two heterosexual individuals? When you evaluate your school's sex education materials and find some that are objectionable, you might be able to get them removed on the basis that they violate the penal code. Call your local police, sheriff's department, or district attorney's office for information about the penal code in your state. Another source for information might be local groups such as Citizens Against Pornography, Citizens for Decency Through Law, or the American Family Association.

D. BECOME INFORMED ABOUT YOUR LOCAL SCHOOL DISTRICT

If you were going to drive through a foreign country that you had never visited before, you would need some basic information before proceeding. You would need a passport (which represents permission to enter), a road map (which guides you through the country), a copy of the traffic laws (to make sure you drive properly), and a driver's license which is valid in that country (which would allow you to drive in that country). Without these items, you would get lost and possibly end up in jail.

The analogy of traveling in a foreign country applies to your interaction with the public schools.

1. Discover the Procedures in Your School District

Before you proceed, you need to find out the school's rules for gaining access to their information and personnel. How are things done within the system? If you have a friend who works in the district, ask some preliminary questions about how curriculum decisions are made and the expected ways in which questions or concerns are raised. This may help you to get started without "red flags of alarm" going up at this stage. Read Appendix B to see how people involved in the battle over sex education view each other.

Call the central office in your school district and ask about the appropriate ways to gain information about curriculum policy or class room practice. For your convenience, use the form in Appendix H when asking questions about the official procedures in the school district. Be sure to make a note of the person who furnished you with the information and whether they are citing official rules or informal procedure.

Appendix B
Differing Views: What People Think of Each Other

Appendix H
Locating Information in the District

2. Find Out About the Structure of Your School District

Many parents do not realize that a school district is comprised of more than teachers, principals, students, and school buildings. Finding out about the structure and personnel will help you identify the various people with whom you must interact, and to whom you must ultimately appeal.

Most school districts have a personnel directory which lists the names of teachers, nurses, counselors, principals, schools, directors, superintendents, and trustees. Try to obtain a current directory from the district's central office. Realize that many school districts are reluctant to release the directory to the public because it might contain the home addresses and phone numbers of school personnel. If you have a friend who works in the district, you might be able to borrow a directory. Sometimes you might be asked to pay for a copy of the directory. Even if you obtain a directory, you will need to find out the area of responsibility of various school personnel, so use the form in Appendix I.

If you are unable to obtain a directory, then call the district office. Ask for the names of certain key people (use the form in Appendix I to find out the questions you need to ask).

Realize that as you begin to inquire about this information, some staff members will begin to assume that you are a troublemaker. Try to defuse any suspicions as much as possible. Use Appendix C for tips on how to reduce the likelihood of creating problems at this stage of the investigation. Getting more than one person to make the calls is helpful.

Appendix I
School District Information

Appendix C
Tips for Gathering Information by Phone

3. Find Out About Sex Education in Your School District

Once you have found out about the proper procedure for obtaining information and from whom to obtain it, your next step is to obtain information about your school district's sex education program. Many parents have already found out something about what is being taught in their child's classes, and that is why they are embroiled in a battle with the school. Sometimes it is what the parents read in their child's biology text. Maybe it was a written assignment that the student had to complete, and the parent accidentally found it in the child's stack of school books. However, a passage in a textbook or an assignment that must be completed by a student is not all that the school has to offer. Possibly the school has some good materials. Maybe it has some bad items, and the principal might not even be aware of it. Regardless of what circumstances face the parent, it is important to have a systematic approach to finding out about the school's sex education program.

Sex education might be labelled as such, but sometimes it is called "family life." Sometimes it is offered as a particular course, and at other times it is a special 1-3 week program. Even if it a separate course or program, sex education is also dealt with in many other courses such as homemaking, biology, health, communicable diseases, etc.

In order to find out what your school district teaches, use the form in Appendix J. When gathering answers, ask for documentation. If you are told something has to be taught, ask for evidence. Also, ask for copies of the course content, objectives, required readings, and supplemental materials.

Anticipate that school personnel will become defensive. (See Appendix B and C for how school personnel might respond.) If they say that parents may only see the materials during the parental preview that is held once a year, don't settle for that answer. Find out the school policies that permit citizens and taxpayers to gain access to information about the schools. However, don't be obnoxious when demanding the information. Always be courteous and persistent. Sometimes, people are more successful in obtaining the answers by meeting personally with the school officials in charge of sex education.

Appendix J
The School's Sex Education Program

Appendix B
Differing Views: What People Think of Each Other

Appendix C
Tips for Gathering Information by Phone

E. FIND OUT WHERE ABSTINENCE EDUCATION IS OFFERED ELSEWHERE

If you have not already interacted with school officials in carrying out the above steps described, you eventually will. You will probably sense that you are considered an outsider. Eventually, when you propose that the schools teach abstinence education, you will discover that some people not only consider you to be an outsider, but they suddenly consider you to be a lunatic fundamentalist!

Therefore, before you go much further, find out what other schools in your area teach abstinence education, as well as the extent to which it is offered across the country. It will sound impressive to say "Abstinence education is required in the states of California, Illinois, Indiana, and Washington, etc.. The *Sex Respect* curriculum is being taught in 500 school districts (find out the current number)." Still, some officials will be more impressed when they hear that school districts nearby have adopted abstinence education.

At this point, you will need to do some homework.

1. Call or Write the Publishers of Abstinence Curricula (see list in Appendix W).

Appendix W
Publishers of Abstinence Education Materials

Ask for the list of all states, cities, and school districts that have purchased or adopted their curricula, particularly the districts in your state or region. Ask for particular names, addresses, phone numbers, and organizations so that you can then call those schools yourself.

While you are on the phone, ask for multiple copies of their promotional literature and order forms. You will use these in your promotional packet at a later stage.

Also consider purchasing a copy of the curricula and their promotional videos (see list in Appendix BB). Having an abstinence curricula or video on hand is helpful when recruiting community support. If you wait too long to place an order for these items, they might arrive too late for your purpose. Some publishers will allow you to review a curriculum without charge for 30 days—you will be responsible for the return postage.

Appendix BB
Audiovisual Resources For Adults on Teenage Sexuality

2. Call or Write the Schools in Your State or Region That Have Adopted Abstinence Curricula.

Obtain information that will help convince your own school personnel that other school districts are sold on the abstinence approach. Use the form in Appendix K to know what information to obtain from school districts which have adopted abstinence education. Be sure to make several photocopies of the form before you begin to fill it in.

Appendix K
Abstinence Programs Elsewhere in Your Region

3. Keep the Completed Forms in Your Files for Future Use When You Are Building Your Case for Abstinence Education.

F. FIND OUT ABOUT TEXTBOOKS

One textbook contained erroneous and biased information about abortion in a section on birth control. The school district had passed a policy stating that instruction on contraception would not be given unless the parents requested it. The administration was caught in a bind—to allow the teachers to teach that section would violate the policy. On the other hand, to forbid the teaching of the section would interfere with academic freedom—an issue that had been recently raised by a teacher's union. So the administration proposed that the board exempt the course (which was an elective class) from the policy. When parents objected, the administration claimed that the law would not allow them to tell the teachers not to teach what was in the state adopted textbook. When asked which law forbade that action,no law was produced.

Because textbooks are approved by the state, they have credibility and are difficult to challenge. Who is the parent to question the "professionals"? The higher the authority, the more weight a statement carries. So the parents must again keep in mind that they are responsible for their children's education. They are the consumers of a product for which they pay dearly. They must be concerned about this crucial issue of textbooks.

Many teachers omit sections of textbooks because they prefer a different approach or do not have enough time to complete an entire text. However, when a textbook includes objectional or inappropriate information, the school district's attitude will often be, "if it is in the book, it must be taught."

Textbooks are of special importance in Texas and California since these two states are the largest purchasers of textbooks. Textbook publishers will write books that appeal to this large market. The rest of the nation will have the same selection of books offered to these two states. In Texas, the State Board of Education approves a proclamation submitted by the Commissioner of Education which includes the required specifications for each subject area. The board appoints a state textbook committee that chooses books to recommend to the board for adoption.

Bringing about change in textbooks is a long-term process. Since books are used for six years or more, this is a very important area for parents to influence. Although members of textbook committees usually are required to be teachers or professionals, the public has the opportunity to be involved in the process. Parents must be committed to study and evaluate the books that are submitted for state adoption. Then, there must be those who will travel to the state capital to testify at textbook hearings. At the local level, individuals must be willing to study and evaluate the state adopted books and testify at local hearings.

Since the textbook issue is a complicated one and requires a long term effort, this manual cannot adequately deal with the subject. We recommend that you contact Mel Gabler, Educational Research Analysts (See Appendix AA), for information on how to get involved in the textbook process.

Appendix AA
Books to Guide Parents

3

EVALUATE YOUR SCHOOL DISTRICT'S SEX EDUCATION PROGRAM

The previous step in this handbook advised you to find out what sex education your school district offers. Possibly you have had the opportunity to see some of the materials, either by attending a parental preview, by seeing your child's textbook, or by getting handouts of certain items from the director of sex education.

BASIC STEPS

If you are working alone or under severe time constraints, it may not be possible to evaluate your school district's total program. Instead, focus on the one portion of the program which aroused your interest in the first place. Find out all you can about that area, then evaluate it in light of the criteria in section C of this chapter.

A. ARRANGE TO EXAMINE THE SEX EDUCATION MATERIALS

Regardless of how much you have been able to see by this point, you need to begin a careful review of all materials, policies, etc. Set up an appointment with the director of sex education. State the purpose of the meeting on the phone so that the person will have the materials available at the meeting. Find out in advance if you will be able to check out materials from their office or obtain photocopies. If not, be prepared to spend considerable time in the office reviewing the material. Also, bring along two or three other parents in order to get multiple reactions.

Before going to the meeting, carefully study the criteria listed at the end of this chapter. The criteria will help you determine the characteristics of an effective sex education program and the characteristics of a harmful one.

If you are only allowed to review the materials in the office and you cannot check them out or get photocopies, then you will have to take careful notes. While seeing a film, use the evaluation form in Appendix L.

Appendix L
Evaluating Your School's Sex Education Program

Beyond reviewing materials, obtain permission to sit in on sex education classes. Take notes during the class and file them with your other information on sex education materials.

B. WRITE A CRITIQUE OF THE DISTRICT'S SEX EDUCATION PROGRAMS AND POLICIES

1. Critique the Program Materials.

After previewing the sex education materials and writing notes about the materials, you are now ready to write a critique of the program's good and inappropriate features. Though your written critique may be lengthy, it will be important in helping you and other parents to understand what needs to be accomplished in your school district.

One of the problems you might find in putting together this critique is "How do I go about organizing all the information that I have accumulated and integrating it with my critique?" Take advantage of the existing organization found within the school system.

- If the district classifies its sex education programs and materials by grade level, then follow that pattern.
- If your school district classifies sex education materials by course content, then use that as your pattern.
- If your school district classifies sex education according to topics (or "essential elements"), then use that pattern.
- If your school district uses a combination of these patterns, then you use a combination of these patterns.
- If there is not a clear pattern describing the program in your district, then follow the pattern in the criteria listed at the end of this chapter.

Next to each item listed as a part of the district's sex education program, write an assessment based on the criteria in Appendix J of this manual and the notes that you took during the review of the materials. Avoid simply saying "It is good." Instead, say **why** it is good. For example, "The unit on how to say no to sexual pressure is excellent because it equips students with the practical skills to resist peer pressure." Instead of saying that something is bad, be specific. For example, "The film entitled 'John and Sally Go On a Date' is inappropriate for fifth graders because it uses vulgarity, it presents the view that sexual activity is normal on dates, and it contributes to a teenager's disrespect for authority figures." Be sure to mention any items that might violate the state's penal code (i.e., "The film takes a neutral stand on sodomy which is illegal in our state").

Besides following the advice above, include a sheet that answers these questions about a program:

1. What is the purpose of the program?
   Is it in writing?
   Is the purpose valid?

2. What is the goal of the program?
   How well is the goal being met?
   What evidence exists to prove the goal is being met?
3. What is the rationale for the program?
   Does the need still exist?
   Is the need valid?
4. What evidence exists that shows success in meeting the need?
   Is the evidence valid, or is it based on feelings (i.e., "the teachers like it")?
   What methods were used to measure success?

Sometimes these questions can help decide if a program—good or bad—is truly needed in a school at all.

2. Critique the Policies and Procedures.

Keep in mind that you might not find objectionable materials in a program, but that doesn't mean the program is automatically a good one. Be sure to note whether a policy upholds the right type of program, whether there is a forum for parental involvement, and whether values are taught when the facts are presented. On the other hand, as you put together the information that you've gathered, you may realize some reasons why your district has less than desirable programs or materials. You may find that a policy or procedure is inadequate or that no clear policy exists.

One group of parents described what they learned about their district policies, guidelines and programs:

> "The district did not have a policy which specifically covers the area of sex education. Specific guidelines for selection of sex education materials and programs did not exist. A written rationale and stated goals did not exist. As a result, there was not an adequate procedure for notifying parents about programs. The teachers had too much freedom in choosing whom to invite in as speakers. There was no opportunity for parental input in the selection of materials and programs. The school board did not review or approve all the materials. Although the P.T.A. council did review materials, they were not required to notify their membership that the materials existed or where they could be reviewed. Nor were parents provided with selection criteria. The school board was not required to approve the materials although they may have seen some of them.
>
> "The district's program included a presentation of facts in areas such as human growth and reproduction and communicable disease. However, a standard of premarital abstinence was not upheld. The physical, psychological, and emotional consequences of premarital sexual activity were not discussed."

Do not simply critique the small points of a school's sex education program. Carefully evaluate the district's written policies and guidelines regarding sex education. You also need to critique the perspective that is taught to teachers and is therefore reflected in the classroom regardless of whether the materials are appropriate.

Use Appendix J as you work on your critique of the school district's policies and guidelines. Also, preview Chapter 4 of this manual before preparing your critique.

Appendix J
The School's Sex Education Program

C. CRITERIA FOR EVALUATING YOUR SCHOOL'S SEX EDUCATION PROGRAM

NOTE: The following criteria pages may be reproduced and distributed to parents helping in your evaluation process.

ROLE OF PARENT IN THE SCHOOL'S DECISION-MAKING PROCESS

BENEFICIAL CHARACTERISTIC	HARMFUL CHARACTERISTIC
1. Involves parents in setting school policies and guidelines about sex education	1. Does not involve parents in the process of setting school policies and guidelines
2. Involves parents in the review and selection of all sex education materials	2. Does not involve parents in reviewing and selecting sex education materials
3. Allows parents ample time to preview all sex education materials before use in the classroom	3. Does not allow parents to preview all sex education materials, or gives short notice about preview dates
4. Gives parents the option to reject materials	4. Does not allow parents the option to reject materials
5. Requires written parental consent to "opt in" so that children may participate in sex education, not placing any stigma on parents or child by asking them to "opt out"	5. Only allows parents the choice to "opt out" their children from sex education, thereby subjecting their child to potential ridicule from peers
6. Provides adequate notification, i.e., mails letter, and places notice in newsletter	6. Notification only in form of slip sent home without requiring parental signature.

ROLE OF PARENT IN THE EDUCATION OF THEIR CHILDREN

BENEFICIAL CHARACTERISTIC	HARMFUL CHARACTERISTIC
Curriculum has a clear-cut method of parental involvement in the education of their child. Examples: — parent training workshop — parent workbook — parent-teen communication worksheets to be taken home daily	Curriculum has no clear method of parental involvement, or vaguely tells the student to discuss the subject with parents

PORTRAYAL OF PARENT IN THE CURRICULUM

BENEFICIAL CHARACTERISTIC	HARMFUL CHARACTERISTIC
1. Parent is portrayed respectfully	1. Parent is portrayed disrespectfully
2. Parent is viewed as a valuable source of information	2. Parent is viewed as ignorant or inhibited or is not mentioned
3. Parent is viewed as the person to turn to in a crisis	3. Student is given other sources to turn to in a crisis
4. Students who bring up sensitive or controversial issues such as masturbation, homosexuality, etc., are told to discuss the issues with parents	4. Controversial issues are discussed openly; guest speakers endorsing homosexuality, etc., are permitted in classroom; students are referred to community agencies instead of to parents
5. When asked about the law, points out that though the law allows certain acts, harm can result; moral as well as legal aspects are considered; students are referred to parents for help	5. Endorses laws such as students' right to an abortion without parental consent or notification, and a student's right to obtain contraceptives without parental consent

MORAL PERSPECTIVE

BENEFICIAL CHARACTERISTIC	HARMFUL CHARACTERISTIC
1. Value-based	1. Attempts to be value-free or value-neutral or non-judgmental
2. Believes in moral absolutes	2. Believes morals are relative
3. Presents views that are consistent with Judeo-Christian values (though it does not teach religion)	3. Views violate traditional Judeo-Christian values
4. Principles are used to teach what is right	4. Avoids the words "right" and "wrong" when teaching the students about choices
5. Points out the right options	5. Presents various options on equal footing and leaves the choice to the student
6. Does not allow students to vote on what is right	6. Lets peers vote on what options to follow
7. Realizes that adolescents do not use adult reasoning, and therefore guides teens to make right choices	7. Treats adolescents like adults

SEXUAL DEVELOPMENT

BENEFICIAL CHARACTERISTIC	HARMFUL CHARACTERISTIC
1. Distinguishes between animals and humans	1. Does not differentiate between animals and humans
2. Teaches that there are emotional and physical stages of life, including childhood, adolescence, and adulthood	2. Assumes that adolescents are like adults
3. Protects the latency period (childhood) and keeps it innocent*	3. Too much too soon, particularly at the elementary level
4. When presenting anatomy and physiology, separates the audience by gender	4. Coed setting regardless of topic
5. Uses proper terminology for anatomy and physiology	5. Uses slang, or encourages students to use slang
6. Protects natural inhibition toward the subject of sexuality	6. Arouses curiosity, promotes openness
7. Teaches modesty	7. Takes a neutral stand on dress and behavior
8. Does not arouse student's sense of pleasure	8. Pleasure oriented (i.e., points out erogenous zones)

* See guidelines by Educational Guidance Institute in Appendix AA.

VIEW TOWARD ABSTINENCE

BENEFICIAL CHARACTERISTIC	HARMFUL CHARACTERISTIC
1. Defines abstinence as restraint from all sexual activity	1. Simply defines abstinence as non-penetration; leaving the idea that anything goes, i.e., anal sex, oral sex, mutual masturbation and other sexual activity
2. Uses the words "premarital abstinence" as the standard to uphold	2. If abstinence is discussed at all, avoids the absolute standard of "premarital abstinence." Instead it uses "wait until you are ready," "postpone sexual involvement," and "psycho-social maturity"

VIEW TOWARD ABSTINENCE ***continued***

BENEFICIAL CHARACTERISTIC	HARMFUL CHARACTERISTIC
3. Premarital abstinence is presented as a positive behavior	3. Abstinence is presented in neutral terminology (such as "abstinence is okay") or in negative terms (it is "old-fashioned" or it is a "joke")
4. Abstinence is presented as attainable	4. Abstinence is viewed as unrealistic
5. The statistics about the high percentage of teens who are abstaining are communicated	5. It is assumed that "everyone" or "most people" are doing it
6. "Secondary virginity" is taught	6. It is assumed that once a teen has had one experience, he or she is "sexually active" and won't stop
7. Abstaining teens are viewed as popular	7. Sexually active teens are viewed as popular
8. Sex drive is taught as controllable	8. Sex drive is taught as uncontrollable
9. Respect for self and others is taught	9. Uncommitted, premarital sex is considered acceptable as long as the "two people care about each other"
10. Respects the student's privacy about self	10. Asks the student to disclose personal information about feelings and behavior
11. Teaches skill building techniques of saying no	11. No help is offered to students on how to handle peer pressure

CONSEQUENCES OF PROMISCUITY

BENEFICIAL CHARACTERISTIC	HARMFUL CHARACTERISTIC
1. Discusses the short-range and long-range psychological freedoms that accompany chastity	1. Says that "if it feels good, do it," ignoring the short-range and long-range psychological problems resulting from promiscuity
2. Shows that marital fidelity is beneficial	2. Takes a neutral or permissive stand toward adultery

SEXUALLY TRANSMITTED DISEASES

BENEFICIAL CHARACTERISTIC	HARMFUL CHARACTERISTIC
1. Defines "safe sex" and "responsible sex" only in terms of premarital abstinence and marital fidelity	1. Defines "safe sex" and "responsible sex" in terms of contraceptive usage
2. Presents a complete review of all sexually transmitted diseases	2. Covers only a few diseases
3. Shows the epidemic status of certain sexually transmitted diseases	3. Takes lightly the epidemic status of sexually transmitted diseases
4. Shows the tragedy of having a sexually transmitted disease	4. Mentions famous people who have had sexually transmitted disease, not telling the tragic consequences. Openly shows teens talking about having a STD without embarrassment
5. Shows the incurability of certain types of sexually transmitted diseases	5. Takes lightly the incurability of certain diseases, or talks about the importance of regular visits to a clinic
6. Points out that certain STDs are asymptomatic	6. Does not stress that certain STDs are asymptomatic and can be transmitted unknowingly
7. Points out that certain STDs lead to sterility	7. Does not stress that certain STDs can lead to sterility
8. Discusses various means of AIDS transmission and teaches avoidance of those behaviors	8. Teaches "protect yourself," not "just say no"
9. Emphasizes the failure rate of condoms in preventing the spread of sexually transmitted diseases	9. Promotes condom usage by suggesting their use, downplaying the failure rate

VARIOUS LIFESTYLES

BENEFICIAL CHARACTERISTIC	HARMFUL CHARACTERISTIC
1. If questions about anal sex are asked, tells about sodomy laws in some states; mentions that sodomy can cause physical harm; refers student to parent	1. Accepts sodomy as a normal practice, or treats it neutrally

VARIOUS LIFESTYLES ***continued***

BENEFICIAL CHARACTERISTICS	HARMFUL CHARACTERISTICS
2. If questions about deviant behavior are asked, mentions the physical and psychological harms; advocates that persons with such behaviors should seek help	2. Does not treat deviant behaviors or lifestyles as harmful
3. Heterosexual intercourse presented as the norm, others are deviant	3. Kinds of sex (i.e., vaginal, anal, oral) are spoken of on the same level

CONTRACEPTION

BENEFICIAL CHARACTERISTIC	HARMFUL CHARACTERISTIC
1. Does not promote contraceptive usage among unmarried teens	1. Advocates that sexually active teens should use contraceptives
2. If contraceptives are discussed, then the risks and failure rates are presented, particularly as they pertain to teens	2. Does not include a discussion of the harms of certain contraceptives, and minimizes the failure rates
3. Discussions of contraceptives are in the context of marriage and family (husband and wife)	3. Discussions of contraceptives are in context of partner, date, boys, girls, etc.
4. Does not demonstrate contraceptive methods or show contraceptive kits	4. Provides instruction on kinds, methods, and how-to's of contraception
5. Respects religious views that oppose contraceptive use	5. Scoffs at religious views objecting to contraceptive use

ABORTION

BENEFICIAL CHARACTERISTIC	HARMFUL CHARACTERISTIC
1. Points out that certain contraceptives can serve as abortifacients (i.e., IUD)	1. Does not point out abortive qualities of certain contraceptives
2. Points out that interception ("morning after pill") is abortion, not contraception	2. Does not disclose the truth about interception

ABORTION ***continued***

BENEFICIAL CHARACTERISTICS	HARMFUL CHARACTERISTICS
3. Does not present abortion as an acceptable alternative to an unwanted pregnancy	3. Presents abortion as an acceptable option for an unwanted pregnancy, or refers to it as a birth control method
4. Points out the potential physical and psychological harms of abortion	4. Downplays or denies the physical and psychological harms of abortion
5. Defines abortion as taking the life of an unborn child; fetal development discussed	5. Defines abortion as termination of pregnancy; no mention of unborn baby

STERILIZATION

BENEFICIAL CHARACTERISTIC	HARMFUL CHARACTERISTIC
Emphasizes the permanence of sterilization	Presents sterilization as a favorable option; talked about as beneficial for financial hardships and world overpopulation

ADOPTION

BENEFICIAL CHARACTERISTIC	HARMFUL CHARACTERISTIC
Presents adoption as a positive option to consider if facing an unwanted pregnancy, emphasizing what is best for the child	Ignores or downplays adoption as an option to consider when facing an unwanted pregnancy; talks about reasons not to have a baby; focuses primarily on the mother, making abortion seem advantageous

SOCIAL DEVELOPMENT

BENEFICIAL CHARACTERISTIC	HARMFUL CHARACTERISTIC
1. Sets standards and describes responsibilities of friendship	1. Doesn't set standards
2. Promotes appropriate group activities rather than pairing	2. Concentrates on one-to-one relationships
3. Helps students to set high standards for the type of people they will date	3. Doesn't discuss standards
4. Suggests appropriate activities for teens on dates	4. Assumes that teens can choose any type of activities
5. Teaches respect between teens	5. Assumes that behaviors are acceptable as long as both people consent

MARRIAGE

BENEFICIAL CHARACTERISTIC	HARMFUL CHARACTERISTIC
1. Uses the word "marriage" and defines it as a life-time commitment	1. Uses the terms "monogamy" or "long-term relations," not "marriage"
2. Presents marriage in favorable terms	2. Marriage has a neutral or negative connotation
3. Marriage is defined as a legal commitment as well as a social and spiritual commitment	3. Live-in relationships are discussed; refers to partners
4. Defines marriage in terms of husband and wife, and spouses	4. Avoids the words "husband" and "wife;" Uses "partners" or "couple"
5. Sexual intercourse within marriage is presented in positive terms	5. No discussion of saving sexual intercourse until marriage; premarital sex is acceptable
6. Unitive and procreative aspects off sexual intercourse are presented as favorable in marriage	6. Pleasure-oriented view of sexual intercourse
7. Marital fidelity is stressed; adultery is presented as harmful to all parties involved	7. Adultery is considered as normal and having no consequences, or treated neutrally
8. Commitment is discussed	8. Trial marriages and live-in situations are discussed without regard to consequences

FAMILY

BENEFICIAL CHARACTERISTIC	HARMFUL CHARACTERISTIC
1. Defined as a blood or legal relationship	1. Defined simply as people living in same household
2. Presented as an important unit in the development of children	2. Society is given greater emphasis than family in child nurture
3. Teaches that commitment, love, and responsibilities are important family traits to develop; discourages divorce and encourages conflict resolution	3. Emphasizes the disintegration of the family as inevitable and irreversible; Does not mention the need for conflict resolution

FAMILY ***continued***

BENEFICIAL CHARACTERISTICS	HARMFUL CHARACTERISTICS
4. Presented as valuable resource to turn to in all situations	4. Talks about other sources to turn to before family
5. The presence of children is presented in favorable terms	5. Children are considered a burden
6. Traditional family roles are respected	6. Ridicule of traditional family roles
7. Teaches respect of the nuclear and extended family	7. Implies disrespect for family members
8. Teaches respect for family rules	8. Greater emphasis is given to the individual's own preferences
9. Respects the privacy and lives of the student's family	9. Asks student to disclose personal information about family

HUMAN REPRODUCTION

BENEFICIAL CHARACTERISTIC	HARMFUL CHARACTERISTIC
1. Discusses human reproduction in proper terminology	1. Uses slang
2. Presents the unborn child as a human being	2. Does not consider an embryo or fetus to be a human life
3. Discusses bonding between mother and child that occurs during pregnancy	3. Discusses bonding only after birth
4. Discusses the importance of the husband's emotional support during pregnancy	4. Does not consider the husband/father's emotional support for pregnant women and for unborn baby
5. Emphasizes the importance of good prenatal care	5. Says that limited amounts of alcohol, etc., won't harm the unborn child; Fear tactics used, which leads the person toward choosing abortion

PARENTING

BENEFICIAL CHARACTERISTIC	HARMFUL CHARACTERISTIC
1. Emphasizes the joy of having children	1. Views children as a burden
2. Emphasizes that parenting involves maturity	2. Stresses that a teen-ager might not have the maturity to be a good parent, thus abortion is acceptable
3. Shows the importance of parents spending "quantity" and "quality" time with their children; recognizes the dangers of enrolling small children in day care centers on a full-time basis	3. Discusses only "quality" time; implies that two parents can work full-time and be adequate parents by spending a few "quality" moments with their children
4. Does not advocate limiting family size	4. Emphasizes overpopulation, the goal of zero population growth

SAFEGUARDS IN DESIGN

BENEFICIAL CHARACTERISTIC	HARMFUL CHARACTERISTIC
1. Has clearly stated policies, guidelines, and objectives consistent with the beneficial criteria listed above	1. Has policies, guidelines, and objectives consistent with the harmful criteria listed above; or, policies, guidelines and objectives are vague or subjective, i.e., "teach students to be responsible," but "responsible" is never defined; i.e., "promote the well-being of the student," but "well-being" is never defined
2. Upholds the highest standards	2. Does not uphold the highest standards
3. No loopholes	3. Has loopholes, thereby allowing teachers to present harmful materials in the class
4. Has a consistent perspective	4. Contains mixed messages, i.e., "abstinence is best, but if you're going to be sexually active, use contraceptives"

SAFEGUARDS IN DESIGN ***continued***

BENEFICIAL CHARACTERISTICS	HARMFUL CHARACTERISTICS
5. The person leading the class and who serves as the source of information is the teacher or nurse	5. Students conduct the course, serve as counselors, are portrayed as authorities, etc.
6. Teacher must be a model of high moral conduct	6. Teacher's moral conduct is considered irrelevant
7. Has a built-in method of assessing student understanding of factual information	7. Does not test for factual comprehension
8. Has a method of assessing students' shift toward positive moral views, yet does not ask for students' names	8. Not concerned about assessing students' shift toward positive moral views; If students' views are polled, asks for names
9. Willingness on the part of the school to seek out the best methodology and materials, and make improvements in order to achieve the above criteria	9. Leans toward trends in methodology rather than effectiveness
10. Upholds the law (i.e., laws against sodomy, pornography, etc.)	10. Includes material that violates or ridicules the law

In addition to the criteria listed above, see the standards listed in section V. C. of *Has Sex Education Failed Our Teenagers? A Research Report* (available from Focus on the Family). Other useful resources are:

1. Judith Echaniz, *When Schools Teach Sex* (see Appendix AA for details).
2. Educational Guidance Institute, *Curriculum Guidelines for Grade Levels* (see Appendix AA for details).

4

DECIDE WHAT NEEDS TO BE DONE IN THE SCHOOLS

BASIC STEPS

If you are facing a deadline to deal with a specific problem, focus your efforts in two areas:

1. What needs to be done to remove the objectionable material or procedure? Be sure you can clearly articulate what is wrong with the present practice.
2. What positive materials or procedures should be used instead? Be sure you are not locked into a negative approach. Be prepared to offer positive alternatives.

After writing an evaluation of materials, procedures and policies in your school district, the next step is to decide what needs to be done to assure that the district provides an excellent sex education program.

Eliminating objectionable materials is a worthy goal, but it does not guarantee that they will not be replaced with equally objectionable materials. Assuring a good film on reproduction at one grade level does not affect what happens in other grades and classes. As long as we direct our efforts toward controlling what happens in the classroom, we are ignoring the source of the problem. We will settle one problem in one area and a problem will surface in another area. We will wear ourselves out putting out brushfires while the raging fire threatens the entire forest. Our children will move on through school and graduate, and few parents will be left to fight the brushfires—if they are even aware of them.

In almost any public school situation, the root cause of any material or procedure is law or policy. Law and policy at the state or local level controls everything from the school calendar to curriculum and textbook content. The bottom line is that someone will decide policy. We must affect policy and influence policy-makers.

A. PROPOSE A GOOD POLICY FOR THE SCHOOL DISTRICT

A good policy lays a foundation. It communicates a clear message to the school staff, students, and community. It sets a standard for the district staff and students. It reflects the moral philosophy of the board. It excludes the "bad" while allowing the "good" curricula, programs, materials, and guest speakers. While it would be beneficial to get a particular curriculum adopted, it is far better to get a good policy passed. The curriculum could become outdated, altered to reflect a particular teacher's perspective, or rejected by newly hired staff. Policy changes require board action at a public meeting.

The importance of policies cannot be overstated. They are, in essence, the law that governs the operation of the school district. As stated previously, curricula, staff, and guidelines may vary, but changes in policy require a board vote. Even if your state has a law, there is a need for a policy to reflect how the law will be carried out in your district.

A policy provides for a certain amount of control. Too much control is too restrictive, but too little control leaves too much discretion to the administration, department head, or individual teacher. The following are suggestions for what an abstinence-based sex education policy should do:

- set and uphold the standard of premarital chastity and fidelity in marriage, advocating "abstinence from premarital sexual activity" (This latter phrase is important because when some groups apply abstinence to sexual intercourse only, leaving the option of all other forms of sexual activity, i.e., sodomy, oral copulation and mutual masturbation within their definition of abstinence. Some of the more progressive educators refer to these as "outercourse.");
- cover all instructional programs, materials, and speakers;
- be age-appropriate and respect latency period (for guidelines on what is age-appropriate at each grade level, obtain the material from Educational Guidance Institute listed in Appendix AA.);
- provide for parental permission, parental review, and parental right to exclude a child;
- eliminate desensitizing materials/programs and respect students' modesty;
- not allow explicit discussion of deviant sexual acts;
- eliminate mixed messages;
- not present homosexuality as an acceptable or normal lifestyle;
- provide for a program adoption process which provides an opportunity for community input.

Appendix AA
Books to Guide Parents

After deciding what a policy should do, write a first draft. Have others read it and tell you their interpretation. Pay close attention to terminology and context. Examine it for loopholes. How might the opposition interpret it to their advantage?

The policy draft should be compared to current law. Is a deviant sex act defined by law? Is lawful marriage a heterosexual marriage? Does the law make it illegal to engage in sexual activity with a minor? Laws can be used as a basis, but policies can go beyond the law to reflect community desires and standards. There may be complaints about a policy, but they lose their strength when the policy is based on law. For example, if your state is one of the 25 in the U.S. in which sodomy is illegal, presenting homosexuality as acceptable or normal would not be upholding the standard set by law.

In the absence of law, a health standard can be used to write or defend a policy. It is easy to make a case that premarital abstinence is the healthiest choice students can make, physically and emotionally.

B. PROPOSE GOOD GUIDELINES FOR THE SCHOOL DISTRICT

Guidelines are more specific than policies and can establish such things as selection criteria for materials, how parental permission will be obtained, who is responsible for selecting materials, and complaint procedures.

A complaint procedure might include a review committee comprised of parents who would consider any objections and make a recommendation for resolution to the Superintendent. Parents with an objection should be allowed to address the review committee. Parents should be included in the selection process.

Criteria for Evaluating Your School's Sex Education Program (Chapter 3, Section C) can be used to develop guidelines. Some other concerns that should be addressed in sex education guidelines are:

- publicity of the district's intention to adopt new materials and/or programs or to consider policy changes;
- availability of all new programs and materials for parental review prior to adoption;
- opportunity for parental input to the district staff regarding materials and programs prior to adoption;
- opportunity for parental and community input to the school board prior to the adoption of new materials and programs;
- notification to parents of any outside speakers/presentations;
- provisions for separating students by sex in order to protect modesty.

C. PROPOSE A GOOD PROTOCOL FOR THE DISTRICT

A protocol is even more specific than guidelines and might address such issues as how certain subjects are handled in the classroom. An example of a protocol would be a list of recommended answers to questions that students commonly ask. A protocol can provide guidance as to how sensitive questions might be handled. Having a protocol can prevent teachers from going beyond what is necessary to answer the question or giving inappropriate answers. For example, if a student asks, "What is an abortion," a teacher could reply that it is a form of birth control that terminates a pregnancy. A more appropriate answer would be that it is a medically induced procedure that takes the life of the unborn baby.

5

MAKE YOUR CASE IN WRITING

BASIC STEPS

Even if time is severely limited, use the outline below to organize your thoughts and information before you meet with school personnel or officials. Effective preparation is essential to an effective presentation.

Having done your homework thus far and having formulated your particular goal (such as the need for a good policy), you are now ready to develop a case for your proposal. You might think at this point, "But I have already done that. I've written a critique of the program and a good policy for the school district to adopt. Isn't that enough writing?"

What you have done so far is important, but you need a persuasive tool to help you win the support of parents and school officials. You will use your critique and suggested policy in building your "case"–your presentation of why school officials should adopt an abstinence policy and curriculum. Your case needs to be in writing, and from it you can develop talks or other persuasive tools.

A. PUT TOGETHER A CASE

This simply outline will help you effectively move through the key elements of your proposal.

I. The teenage sexuality crisis in your community
II. What the school has attempted to do
   A. What the school is offering
   B. Your evaluation of the school's program (both good and bad features)
III. What needs to be done to improve the school's program
   A. The policy, guidelines, etc. that you are proposing
   B. The recommendation of an abstinence curriculum.
IV. Evidence that your proposal will help to improve the conditions for teenagers
   A. Evidence that abstinence education works
   B. Where abstinence education has been adopted elsewhere in your region
   C. Refuting common objections (refer to section V. B. "Myths About Abstinence Education" in the sex education report)
V. Specific action required and by whom

B. PUT TOGETHER A PROMOTIONAL PACKET

After developing your case in writing, put together multiple sets of a promotional packet that you can give to key decision makers at school, to influential people in the community, and to other people whom you encounter. You will need —

- folders,
- clear photocopies of your case,
- multiple copies of the sex education report,
- order forms for abstinence curricula (available from publishers).

You might also obtain a promotional video (see Appendix BB in this handbook.) and curriculum samples (see Appendix W) to include with your packet.

Even if you don't have the money to invest in all of these items, invite friends, a Sunday school class, a Bible study group, or civic group if they would like to underwrite the cost. Or, it is possible to put together inexpensive promotional packets to distribute to selected school personnel. To reduce the cost, you could loan your packet to one school decision-maker, and then pass it along to others. However, this sharing procedure might be too time consuming and prolong the process of influencing school decision-makers.

On the outside of your packet (folder), place a positive title such as "An Innovative Approach to Reducing Teenage Pregnancy." The first page of the packet should be a cover sheet with information about your group (its name, address, phone number, contact person, and objective). If you are working alone, then put your name, address, and phone number on the outside of the packet. After the cover page, put a letter to school personnel asking them to carefully review the packet. Keep the letter on a positive note. Then include a table of contents. After that, place a written copy of your case. In the pocket of the folder, place a copy of the sex education report and order forms for abstinence curricula.

NOTE: Be sure to type all materials for your packet. Also, make good photocopies. School officials and other community leaders will partly assess the integrity of abstinence education on the basis of your packet.

6

CONTACT THE SCHOOL'S KEY DECISION-MAKERS

BASIC STEPS

If time is limited, it is important that you talk directly with the school person most directly involved in the area of concern and the person with the authority to make the desired change. Be sure that your time constraints do not stampede you into making enemies of concerned people who were inadvertently excluded.

Now you are on your journey to influencing people to adopt your proposal! The first people you will want to interact with are the various decision makers at school.

When parents realize that they must talk face-to-face with school administrators, they often shy away because of feelings of inadequacy. If you feel this way, consider the various levels that Paul went through in order to present his case to governing bodies. In Acts 22-28, Paul appealed—

- first to the Jews,
- then to the Sanhedrin Council,
- then to Felix, the Roman governor,
- then to Festus, his successor,
- then to King Agrippa,
- and finally to Caesar.

Paul had the courage to go through this process because the Lord had told him that he would be a witness for His cause, even in Rome, the seat of the highest ruler of his day. As educated and capable as Paul had been prior to his conversion, he needed to rely on God's guidance when going before these officials. Likewise, you need to draw your strength from the Lord and welcome the opportunity to present your case to the school administration.

A. SET UP APPOINTMENTS

Set up appointments with those people who are involved in the school's decision-making process (i.e., teachers, department heads, directors, etc.). It is wise to start with the lower levels (i.e., teacher) and then move on up through higher levels (i.e., director of sex education). People appreciate the courtesy of being included in discussions about their area of responsibility. Following this pattern also allows the school personnel the chance to activate their system from within. Finally, you don't want school personnel to hear that you are out recruiting support for your proposal before you have presented your ideas directly to them.

In setting up appointments, call the person and ask for a meeting at their office. State the purpose for the meeting by presenting a positive message such as "Because you are involved in addressing the teenage pregnancy problem, I would like to meet with you to share some excellent information and resources that I have come across." Request adequate time for the appointment. If you plan to show a promotional video, then take that into consideration. Be sure to ask the person to arrange for VCR equipment to be there at the meeting.

Explain that one or two other parents will attend the conference with you. We cannot overstate the importance of including others. First, when two or three meet with a school official, their concern is more likely to be taken seriously and less likely to be dismissed with "you're the only parent who believes that way." Also, the other people who attend are helpful in recalling what occurred at the meeting. Finally, by having other parents attend, you are training them to be able to speak with school personnel. These parents, in turn, will develop more confidence in being able to speak up at other meetings.

Before going to the meeting, review the common myths in Appendix B and Appendix P of this handbook.

Appendix B
Differing Views: What People Think of Each Other

Appendix P
Common Arguments and How to Answer Them

B. GO TO THE MEETING

Before going to the meeting, ask friends to pray for you while you are at the meeting.

When you meet with teachers, focus your discussion on issues and materials. Find out from the teachers how much input teachers have in the selection of materials. The information that you gather from teachers can be helpful when meeting with the administration. When meeting with people in administration, focus more on policies and guidelines rather than the minor details.

At the meeting, state who you are and the positive message that you have. If you are working with a group, tell something about your goals and your members. State something positive about the person you are meeting with and something positive about the schools. Share your concern about teenage pregnancy. Stress the commonality you share with the person and the school. Describe your discovery that old approaches to the problem of teenage pregnancy have not worked, but that there are now new approaches that are proving to be highly successful. At that point, show the promotional video on abstinence education (if you have purchased one). Ask for the person's reactions to the video. Then discuss your proposal for the school. Show specific reasons why that particular person would like your proposal (i.e., a health teacher will respond to information about good health). If your school district's program is in conflict with abstinence education, then point out that many schools are abandoning that approach. If you have brought along sample curricula, show them to the person. Let the person know that you would like them to review your packet. If you leave certain materials that you want returned to you, be sure to indicate that you are loaning the items. Agree upon a time span for the person to review the items, and a specific time that you will pick them up. Set up a time to discuss the person's reactions to your promotional packet.

C. PERSUADE PEOPLE TO READ THE SEX EDUCATION REPORT

One of the goals of the conference will be to place *Has Sex Education Failed Our Teenagers? A Research Report* in the hands of the decision-maker. Keep in mind that a person might graciously accept the report from you, but that doesn't guarantee that he or she will read it or, moreover, be influenced by it. So you must carefully plan how to **persuade** the person to read it.

Here are some useful steps that should make the decision-maker **want** to read it.

1. Express appreciation to the decision-maker for taking the time to meet with you.
2. State that you empathize with the many responsibilities which confront the decision-maker.
3. Express your commitment to work with the school in order to help reduce the teenage sexuality problem.
4. If you have gone through the steps of putting together a promotional packet and recruiting support for your cause, then let the school decision-maker know that there are others who feel as you do and want to work with the school.
5. If in the past, you once believed that the pro-contraceptive approach was the right solution, then state that at one time you believed differently. Briefly share why you no longer believe that way. Don't condemn the people who still subscribe to that approach. Instead, indicate that you believe that such people would be surprised if they were to read major studies showing the ineffectiveness of such programs.
6. If your goal is to get objectionable programs removed from the classroom or to prevent the school from adopting the wrong types of programs, then point out four or five major facts that you learned about the objectionable programs. Indicate that by having read the sex education report, you are convinced that the schools need to avoid such programs.

   When you are seated by the decision-maker, mention one of the facts, turn to the sex education report, and **briefly** point out one quote or piece of evidence that supports your statement.

   Sample:

   "After reading this report, I became convinced that comprehensive sex education contributes to teenage promiscuity. Let me show you. Look at these quotes by some of the advocates of sex education who admit that their programs stimulate sexual activity." (Then point to those quotes and read them aloud.)

7. If your goal is to get abstinence education adopted by the school, then point out four or five major facts that you learned about abstinence education. Indicate that by having read the sex education report, you are convinced that the schools need to adopt abstinence education.

   When you are seated by the decision-maker, mention a fact and then turn to the sex education report and **briefly** point out one quote or piece of evidence in favor of abstinence.

   Sample:

   "Most people believe that schools can't teach abstinence because it is the same as teaching religion. But I was glad to know that the Supreme Court has already ruled that abstinence education is **not** an establishment of religion, and that morality **can** be addressed in the classroom." (Then point to that section of the report and read a **brief** portion of it.)

   "I had no idea until I read this report that abstinence education has actually helped to reduce the teenage pregnancy rate. Here, let me show you some of the studies."

8. State that you know that the person will want to have that kind of information and that is why you are leaving the report. Ask when the person would like to meet to discuss the subject further. (The purpose of making a follow-up appointment is to commit the person to exploring the subject further, particularly by reading the report.) Set up a follow-up meeting.

9. To give an added boost in order to move the decision-maker in the direction of teaching abstinence, mention some of the respected professional people in your community who have endorsed abstinence education.

7

RECRUIT COMMUNITY SUPPORT FOR YOUR PROPOSAL

BASIC STEPS

If you have contacted school personnel about your concern, but the response is not positive, then you must seek to enlist additional people to stand with you. When time is of the essence, select the actions from this chapter which you feel best equipped to do successfully.

While attempting to persuade key decision makers, there should be a simultaneous effort to educate the public. Many people have been taken in by trendy but damaging philosophies. Many mothers, out of fear, have had their daughters put on the "pill." Some parents, burdened with their own stress and problems, have given up trying to be parents in any true sense of the word. They may not like the idea of their teens being sexually active, but they think it may be inevitable. They are uninformed about the effects of the "value-free" sex education of the last 20 years, and they are unaware of true abstinence education materials. They may think that abstinence education consists of only telling students "just say no."

Promoting an idea is like selling a product. Make a list of points you want to communicate to the public. Use the media, public forums, and offer speakers to churches and organizations (see media section). Repetition is an important element.

A. PEOPLE TO APPROACH

Develop a list of individuals and groups of people who can be contacted to provide support for your proposal. Individuals and groups to include on your list could include: parents of school children; taxpayers; church leaders and church members; professionals such as doctors, lawyers, therapists, and counselors; leaders of ministries; civic groups; clubs; and elected officials.

B. HOW TO APPROACH GROUPS AND INDIVIDUALS

There are various ways to approach people who could offer the greatest support for your efforts. Some effective means to consider are:

1. Informal conversations with friends, neighbors, and relatives;
2. Personal contact with a friend who is a member of a group;

3. Presentations which include an explanation of your purpose and a showing of a promotional video (refer to Appendices M, N and O);
4. Flyers distributed to targeted groups;
5. Letters to targeted groups;
6. Newsletter articles announcing your proposal;
7. Press releases (see Chapter 8, Work with the Media and Appendix U);
8. Press conference (see Chapter 8, Work with the Media);
9. Radio or television talk show (see Chapter 8, Work with the Media);
10. Paid advertisement on radio, television or newspaper;
11. Public service announcements on radio, television and in newspapers;
12. Letters to the editor of your local newspapers (see Chapter 8, Work with the Media).

Appendix M
Giving a Talk Before an Audience

Appendix N
Useful Verses to Review Before Speaking

Appendix O
Outline of a Sample Talk

Appendix U
Sample Press Releases

C. CHANNEL PUBLIC OPINION BACK TO KEY DECISION-MAKERS

After you have convinced various individuals and groups of the need to support your proposed policy, channel their opinions back into the school system. This process will let the schools' key decision-makers realize that the community is supportive of your proposal. Here are some methods for directing public opinion back into the schools.

1. When giving talks, always specify the action you want people to take.

Consider the timing when asking for action. A telephone campaign is best just prior to anticipated board action. Letters have a greater impact, but require more time.

a. Ask people to call key decision-makers. Provide names and phone numbers.

b. Ask people to write letters to key decision-makers. Provide names and addresses.

c. Distribute a questionnaire at the end of your talk. Allow time for completing and collecting the questionnaire. Tabulate the results of the questionnaire and pass that information along to school personnel.

d. Ask the president or leader of the group to write a letter on behalf of your efforts.

2. Petition Drive

A petition effort can be an effective means of sending a strong message to the school administration and board. If a large number of signatures are needed, the effort should not be undertaken unless a significant number of people are willing to work at the effort.

Failing to get enough signatures after announcing a petition drive would be embarrassing and hurt your efforts. See sample petition in Appendix S. Factors to consider:

a. The purpose should be clear and concise. The petition should not be so complicated that it has to be explained.

b. A significant number of people must be dedicated to the effort.

c. A deadline must be set for completion of the effort

3. Letter-Writing Party

Hold a 5-minute letter-writing party at the end of one of your talks or at the end of a Sunday school class, Bible study, etc. Bring post-cards or paper and envelopes to the meeting. Briefly explain what should be the main thrust of the letters, but have everyone use their own words. Collect the letters and cards so you can mail them.

4. Endorsements

Ask key individuals to endorse your efforts by writing a letter to key decision-makers. Ask that they provide a copy of their letter to you. Ask if their name can be used as an endorser when publicizing your proposals.

D. KEEP THE PUBLIC UPDATED ON YOUR PROGRESS

You should keep supportive people informed about the progress of your work. Also, let them know if additional action is required at strategic times. Finally, inform them about the outcome of your efforts. Some ways to do this are:

1. Keep a list of names and phone numbers of all people who have shown support for your proposal (i.e., friends, those who filled out your questionnaires; people who wrote letters on your behalf; people at your church; etc.) Ask a member of your group to call these people. If you have access to a phone bank, then use it.

2. Place announcements in newsletters.

3. Call in to radio talk-shows to report the progress.

4. A recorded message can be used to provide up-to-date information. Money can be raised to pay for an additional phone line and a recording machine. The machine could provide a 1-3 minute message for calls and also take messages from callers. A sample message might be:

   "The school board will vote on a proposed abstinence sex education policy at a meeting on Monday, January 14th, at 7 p.m. at the district office at 3200 Fairman Road. Plan to be there early in order to get a seat. Speakers will be limited to 3 minutes each. If you want more information or are interested in joining our effort to get the policy passed, please leave your name and number at the sound of the tone."

In some areas, a message line (voice mailbox) can be leased by the month for less than the cost of a regular phone line. The message service allows you to change the message as often as needed and to take messages from the callers. The recording and message retrieval can be done from any phone.

8

WORK WITH THE MEDIA

BASIC STEPS

Read the 'Tips for Media Contacts' below to help prepare yourself for an approach by a reporter.

Consider writing a letter to the editor to express your position.

Newspapers, radio and television can help you communicate your ideas, educate the public and reinforce your position. Sooner or later you will come in contact with the media. Be prepared and learn to work with them to your advantage.

Repeated contact with the media may help them recognize you as a helpful source when an issue arises. You may be asked to make recommendations of persons to interview on related subjects.

A. TIPS FOR MEDIA CONTACTS

1. Have in mind no more than four or five points you wish to communicate, such as the following:
   - Concept of abstinence education
   - Harmful effects of contraceptives on young people
   - Success of abstinence education
   - Failure of contraceptive education
   - Risk of contraceptive use based on failure rates
2. Be positive. It is much better to be "for" something than "against" it. Even if you are fighting against certain materials or procedures, you can relate it in positive terms.
3. Express confidence (not arrogance) in your position. Be sure to keep informed.
4. Be solution-oriented. Bemoaning a problem without suggesting solutions gains nothing.
5. Try to relate an issue to a root cause. Avoid merely dealing with symptoms.
6. Avoid personal attacks. Sometimes completely ignoring the opposition is best. Avoid being inflammatory.

7. Use terms that the average person can be expected to understand. Keep explanations brief. Do not say anything that you are not prepared to back up with facts or easily understood logic.

B. LETTERS TO THE EDITOR

Most newspapers accept letters from their readers and print them in the editorial section. Some will accept lengthier items for a guest column. This is a great opportunity to express your views. The more letters received on a subject from a variety of individuals, the more likely one on the subject will be printed.

Follow these tips in writing to a newspaper:

1. Comply with the standards set forth by the editor such as length (usually one typewritten page or 300 words or less). Letters should be signed and include your name, address and phone number.
2. Submit letters according to the frequency limits established by the paper. For example, many papers will only print one letter a month from each individual.
3. Write concerning a timely or controversial topic, immediately following a related news article, or to bring facts to the attention of the public.
4. Understand that your letter may be edited if it is too long or contains irrelevant information. Avoid including too many statistics, facts, or quotations since a letter to the editor is intended to express "your" opinion. See Appendix T for forms to use in writing letters to the editor.

Appendix T
Sample Letters to the Editor

C. PRESS RELEASES

A press release is an excellent way to communicate information to the public and identify you as a source of information to the news media. It can be used to communicate your position on an issue or let the public know about a special event. Reporters may contact you to make a statement when related issues arise.

1. Writing a Press Release

A press release should begin with a brief title, have a clear purpose and relate "who, what, when, where, and how." It should be double spaced and name a "contact" person at the top of the page. The contact person should be ready and willing to speak to the media. A one-page concise press release is best; it should not be more than two pages. There should be a strong opening with the most important information at the top and less important information toward the end. Paragraph headings can be used. One or two quotes should be included. Use no more than five objectives you wish to communicate. (See sample press release in Appendix U.)

Appendix U
Sample Press Releases

2. Ideas for Press Releases

Purchase an abstinence education video or video series. Then write a press release about the concept of abstinence education, announcing that your group is offering the video presentation to local groups or churches. Identify whom to contact. A brochure about the video could be included. You could charge a small fee for a presentation, gaining some help with expenses and building a fund to purchase other materials. A speaker should be prepared to introduce the video, answer questions, and encourage the audience to become involved in getting good policies into their schools.

A press release can be prepared prior to a board hearing to notify the press that your group plans to address the board.

Your organization can vote on a resolution calling on the school board to adopt an abstinence policy. Include a copy of the resolution with the press release. (See Appendix U.)

3. Where to Send Press Releases

Press releases should be sent to local news media such as daily and weekly newspapers, radio stations, and television stations. Don't overlook special interest publications such as regionally distributed or denominational publications.

A copy of the press release should be sent to:

a. News publications: City desk and assignment reporter
b. Radio: News department and talk show hosts
c. Television: News department and assignment reporter

D. HOLDING A PRESS CONFERENCE

Hold a press conference when you want to draw attention to something important or when there is a sense of urgency. For example, hold a press conference to announce that several organizations endorse a proposed abstinence sex education policy, or that they oppose the current policy or program.

Plan your press conference in advance. Schedule at least three people to speak for up to three minutes. Prepare speakers to answer questions. Important speakers, elected officials, and well-known individuals draw more attention.

Send a press release one week in advance to notify the media of the speakers, time, place, and subject. Do not go into any detail concerning the subject. Call the day before to confirm that the notification was received and to inquire if a reporter will be attending. If a reporter wants to know more, say you will be glad to talk to him or her after the press conference. You want to convey that you have some big news and want to give it to everyone at the same time.

The best time for a press conference is around 10 a.m. so that the news will be in the afternoon paper or evening news. The location should be large enough to accommodate invited press and their equipment. Sometimes a location can be chosen for effect, such as the steps of the school district office. Be sure to consider weather conditions and assure that the space can be used. Invite supporters to attend, but they should not ask questions.

Start the conference on time and keep it short. Open the conference by thanking the press for attending. Then state the purpose of the press conference. After the speakers give their statements, say, "We'd be glad to answer any questions you might have." It is okay to refer questions to any of the speakers. Reporters will probably interview individuals after the conference. After the conference, give reporters a press release, or press packet.

E. TELEVISION

TV interviews are more difficult since you can't use notes. Have a few main objectives. You have the right to inquire what questions you will be asked. Make sure wind is not blowing your hair and clothes, and the sun or light is not glaring in your eyes. You have the right to change the subject. If the question is totally unacceptable, smile pleasantly (don't grin) and remain silent.

Beware of a pregnant pause when the interviewer asks a question and after you answer. An interviewer often remains silent hoping you will continue to talk. The purpose is to get you to expand on the subject. During the time you're trying to fill the silence, you are most likely to say something you do not want on the air. Smile and remain silent.

Do not wear white. Women should wear makeup so they will not look pale. Large flashy jewelry can create a glare. Relax, look pleasant, and avoid staring. Move your head, not just your eyes.

F. TALKING TO REPORTERS

After all that we have heard about the media bias, the idea of being interviewed can be intimidating. Being prepared can help relieve feelings of anxiety. Some basic tips are:

1. Be concise. The more you expand an answer, the more the reporter can pull particular statements out of context. Also, some reporters simply stop listening after a few sentences. They are looking for brief, quotable statements, not lengthy explanations.

2. If a reporter calls unexpectedly, try to determine what he or she wants to know. Ask if you may call back within a short period of time, allowing you to collect your thoughts.

3. List three to five key points that you want to make. Try to pull all questions back to those points or to information supporting those points. Avoid isolated issues that need a long detailed explanation.

4. Have your supporting information at hand. Use a highlighter or a red pencil to mark information, such as statistics, that you want to quickly find.

5. Try to avoid making any statement that could be isolated and taken out of context.
6. Have some strong statements that communicate a clear, positive message. For example,

   "Teenagers need to know the truth that saving sex for marriage is the healthiest choice they can make."

   "Public schools have the responsibility to uphold a high moral and health standard when they teach sex education."
7. Occasionally you can make a point by answering a question with a question. It can help you make a point prior to answering the question, or it can cause the reporter to examine the issue from a different perspective. It can also help you avoid answering a question that doesn't fit the issue. For example, if you are asked if teaching abstinence is teaching morality, you might say, "Does that mean that not teaching it is teaching immorality?" If asked if requiring abstinence to be taught is imposing your values, you could say, "Whose values are being taught now?" It would usually be beneficial to go ahead and answer the question after you've made your point. Don't use this technique too often, and don't do it in a sarcastic or arrogant way.
8. Sometimes a question requires a complicated answer which opens the door to being misquoted. Before answering you could ask the reporter some questions to determine how much he knows. You also might say, "That's a complicated issue; may I give you some background information off-the-record before I answer that question?" You might learn just how interested the reporter really is in understanding the issue. If there is little interest, the reporter will drop it and you will have avoided being misquoted. Otherwise, you've had an opportunity to explain a difficult area.
9. If a press release has been sent, be sure to keep it near the phone along with your supporting information.
10. Anticipate what the opposition will say and address their arguments before they have a chance to present them. Answer in a positive, confident manner.
11. Remember that your comments may be separated from the question when printed, so always be cautious.
12. Humor or sarcasm is not effective and can project the wrong image.
13. You have the right to change the subject during the interview.
14. While you may request that what you say is "off the record," never take it for granted. Remain cautious.

G. RADIO INTERVIEWS

Voice is important when being interviewed on the radio. The first time you hear yourself, you may be shocked. If you are normally very serious and you're nervous about the interview, you may sound monotonous and boring. Loosen up. Use an upbeat voice! Try to imagine how an outgoing, confident friend would speak. After you are introduced and welcomed to the program, the interviewer may say "Good morning." Responding with a friendly, exuberant, "Good morning!" can help give you a good start.

Sometimes when people are nervous, they sound silly or have a silly laugh. If this is the case, you will need to be more serious.

H. NEWS PROGRAMS

A radio interview can be pre-recorded for playing during the news, or it can be live. In either case it usually will be short so what you say is extremely important. If it is pre-recorded, you might be interviewed for five minutes but only two or three sentences will be used. Have two or three points in mind and make strong, clear statements.

I. RADIO TALK SHOWS

Radio talk-show programs can range from 5 to 55 minutes or more with commercial breaks in between. They can be done in the studio or over the phone. It would be easy to conclude that the interviewer just asks questions, and all that is necessary is to know your subject well and be able to answer questions. This is a naive and simplistic view. It is essential that you have a clear idea of what you want to communicate to listeners. It is best to make an outline of key points you want to make. During the commercial breaks, you can make notes of areas you may have left out. Here are some guidelines:

1. Begin with writing out a clear, strong introductory statement. This can be read aloud if you practice reading it as you would say it.
2. Outline a list of points you want to make with supporting information and then put them in order of priority. Focus on the top three to five points and relate your answers and comments back to these points.
3. Have a separate fact sheet containing statistics and other information at hand to answer any questions.
4. Don't get led down a "bunny trail" that goes nowhere or that leads to a debate over a side issue. Sometimes you can say, "What you are really asking is . . ." and then refocus the question. Or, you might say, "That is a complicated issue; we need to look at what is behind it . . ." and then relate it to your main points or other related information.
5. Don't interrupt, call names, or get entangled in useless arguments.

6. While you may want to discuss a problem, it is even more important to discuss possible solutions. Communicate that something positive can be done rather than give the impression we are all at the mercy of the forces and circumstances around us.

J. OTHER WAYS TO WORK WITH THE MEDIA

1. Recommend guests for talk shows. Call or write the station and give them the name of the guest plus other information such as books authored, positions held, etc. It is helpful if you can include a newspaper article, advertisement for a book, book review, etc., to let the station know more about the person.
2. Suggest a story line to a reporter and provide background information. Suggest people the reporter may contact for further information.
3. Notify the media when a controversial or important issue is on a school board agenda. Offer background information. Share with a reporter that there are some unanswered questions and the public is entitled to answers. Give some sample questions.
4. Use the "open-line" offered on some radio talk-shows to express your opinions.

9

SHARPEN YOUR STRATEGY

While you proceed with your plans to influence the community, be aware that some problems might be occurring as a result of your efforts.

A. DEALING WITH OPPOSITION

Someone or some group is bound to oppose your efforts. Therefore, be prepared for opposition before it happens. Hold a brainstorming session to discuss possible opposition. Who is likely to oppose your proposals? Are they organized? How will they oppose you? What arguments are they likely to use? How will you deal with them?

Follow these helpful guidelines in dealing with any opposition:

1. Probably the most important thing you can do in dealing with the opposition is to anticipate their arguments and address them before they have the opportunity to raise objections. Develop a list of possible arguments and answers to them. (See Section V. B. "Myths About Abstinence Education" in ***Has Sex Education Failed Our Teenagers?*** Also refer to "They Say, We Say" in Appendix P of this handbook.)

Appendix P
Common Arguments and How to Answer Them

2. Don't get caught up in a name-calling exchange. If you are called a name, ask the other party to define the term. For example, a reporter may ask you if you are a fundamentalist because your opposition has referred to you that way. Ask, "What is meant by a fundamentalist?" or "What did (the opposition) mean by that term?"

3. Sometimes ignoring the opposition is the best way to handle them. If you ignore them, others may too. However, sometimes they cannot be ignored.

4. Know what your opponents are doing. Are they holding meetings? Writing letters to the editor? Attending school board meetings? If their meetings are open to the public, you can send a few people to monitor their activities.

5. Be cautious. Avoid alerting the opposition to your strategy. Be careful to whom you provide source material. If your name or your group's name has been in the news media, or you have spoken at public meetings, be leery of phone calls seeking information. Someone may be trying to obtain information that can be used against you. Attempt to determine who referred the caller by asking such questions as, "How did you learn about our group?" If an organization is named, ask who made the referral or how they happened to contact the organization. A few questions will probably provide enough information for you to know if the caller is a friend or foe.

B. MAINTAIN CONTACT WITH KEY DECISION-MAKERS

During the time that you have been trying to influence the public, some school decision-makers might become alarmed by negative press coverage, by misinformation that has been spread about you and your organization, and by groups opposing your proposals. To keep decision makers from moving away from your proposal, maintain ongoing calls with them. Inquire about their opinions and awareness of public reaction. Offer to provide additional facts or materials.

C. CONSIDER TIMING OF SCHOOL BOARD ELECTIONS

Since the school board is the key to getting a good policy, consider when the next school board election will be held. If it is in the next several months, your plans can work toward the election. (See chapter 13, "School Board Elections.") If the school board election is a year or more away, then it will not be a major consideration. The election should be included in your long-range goals, especially if the current board is resistant to your proposal.

10

GO BEFORE THE BOARD

The school board is the governing body that votes on policies for the school district. Therefore, you will need to make an appeal to the board to adopt an abstinence education policy.

A. WHO SERVES ON THE BOARD?

The school trustees, or board members, are residents of the school district who have been elected by the voters in that district. They are supposed to represent the parents and citizens in the district. This responsibility includes representing community values. The importance of the school board and of getting to know the members cannot be overstated.

B. THE SCHOOL BOARD'S ROLE

The school board oversees the operation of the district, but does not normally get involved in its everyday operation. The most important role of the board is deciding policy. Other responsibilities of the board are: hiring the superintendent, budget and purchase order approval, conducting personnel hearings and responding to grievances, and textbook approval.

Most board members and superintendents do not have time to thoroughly review every textbook or purchase order brought before them. They depend on the district staff's recommendations. For example, a committee will review and recommend textbooks to the superintendent, who in turn will recommend their adoption to the school board. Since the school board hired the superintendent, they are likely to trust his or her judgment and approve his or her recommendations unless they have reason to do otherwise. They may not be aware that contraceptive methods are being taught.

Rarely are board members aware of the details of programs, methods, or materials. Because it is impossible for the board to know everything related to their district, parents need to become involved. Parents must hold school boards accountable.

BASIC STEPS

If your original goal is simply to have objectionable materials removed from the classroom, you might have already accomplished your goal in the previous steps described in this handbook. However, in some cases such an action may require a board decision. The suggestions in this chapter will help you present your case effectively.

NOTE: Always keep in mind that even if you accomplish the goal of having offensive materials removed, you should try to get a policy enacted that will prevent future occurrence and which promotes the highest standards for all sex education programs. Even if you are successful in getting a teacher, department head, or principal to use abstinence materials, such a victory is very limited and will not ensure that the abstinence approach is permanent. Therefore, the adoption of an abstinence policy is essential to assure that abstinence education is firmly established.

Individual board members bring their view of education and their personal philosophy to their position. For example, a board member who believes that abortion is a woman's right may not object to a textbook that has a pro-abortion bias. This person might willingly vote for a textbook that presents abortion as a birth control method that is safer than childbirth. Nor may the member object if the book avoids significant information such as the physical complications of abortion or the fact that abortion kills the unborn baby. Therefore, it is essential to identify candidates' positions on crucial issues.

C. THE IMPORTANCE OF CITIZEN INTERACTION WITH THE SCHOOL BOARD

Whether you want to be involved in politics or not, someone will represent your family on the school board. If you refuse to concern yourself with the school board, you forfeit your right to complain.

In many areas, only about 5 percent of the registered voters turn out for a school board election. Most parents do not know who their local school board members are or when the school board election is held. Many whose children are not currently in public school believe that they can't or shouldn't vote in school board elections.

D. HOW TO IDENTIFY BOARD MEMBERS' POSITIONS ON THE ISSUES

One of the best ways to determine what school board members believe is to take a survey. Ideally, this should be done prior to every election. However, it can be done at anytime. A survey will not only identify a candidate's position, it will put the person on record as being for or against specific issues. A board member who refuses to work for, support, or vote for a good policy, can be called to account—publicly. For example, if Mr. Smith has gone on record as being against contraceptive education, he can be reminded of it during a board hearing on the adoption of sex education materials. If after the reminder he votes for it anyway, his stance can be publicly exposed then, and again if he runs for re-election. Surveys are one way to keep board members accountable.

E. DEVELOPING A BOARD MEMBER OR CANDIDATE SURVEY

(See Appendix V for a sample survey.)

Appendix V
Sample School Board Candidate Screening Forms

1. Identify Issues

A survey should include questions concerning current issues in the district as well as issues with the potential to become important in the near future. To be well-balanced, candidate surveys should include a variety of issues, including non-controversial ones.

2. Write Questions

After developing a list of issues, write the questions you want candidates to answer. The questions should be as clear and concise as possible. Read them aloud to friends or your group members and ask for their response. If their answers indicate that they are confused, reword your questions. Frame survey questions so the answers show a contrast in the candidates' positions. Sometimes a second question can elicit a clarifying answer.

The terms used in a survey are extremely important. For example, consider the question, "Are you in favor of academic freedom?" Academic freedom is a term usually applied to colleges and universities and refers to the teacher's freedom to decide matters of classroom discussion and materials. Some people believe high school teachers should have "academic freedom," while others believe it should not apply in public schools with minor children. A candidate might answer in favor of academic freedom without realizing the implications for public schools. In general, if the term needs to be explained, it is best not used.

Terms that are commonly known among educators can be used even though some candidates may not be familiar with them. For example, anyone running for school board should understand the difference between the phonics method and the "sight" method of teaching reading. They should have some knowledge about controversial trends such as school-based health clinics and values clarification. (Note: since an occasional candidate will think that a school-based health clinic is the office of the school nurse, we used the term, "school-based medical clinic" in our survey.)

3. Write a Cover Letter

Write a letter to accompany the survey, giving clear directions and a request that the survey be returned as soon as possible. Send the survey to candidates the day following the election filing deadline. Call the district office to obtain the names and addresses of the candidates. Three to five days after sending the survey, call the candidates to confirm that they received the survey. Ask if they intend to complete and return the survey. Explain that you need the survey returned as soon as possible in order to meet a printing deadline. The candidate should be required to sign the survey and you should retain the original copy of the survey in your files.

When calling candidates, be careful not to answer their questions about the survey in such a way as to prejudice their answers. If they are unfamiliar with an issue, refer them to a source, or explain it in a neutral way.

4. Compile and Print Results

Once the surveys are returned, compile and print the information. To avoid embarrassment and legal difficulty, have someone carefully proofread the survey results. Once the survey is printed, it needs as wide a distribution as possible. Some ideas are:

- Circulate the results to churches, organizations, community events, and Christian bookstores.
- Place the results on community bulletin boards.

- Make the results available to groups who publish newsletters.
- Announce the results in a press release to the media.

F. THE VOTING PATTERNS OF THE BOARD

It is helpful to understand the relationship of the board and the administration and to learn how the board functions. To discover these patterns, attend several board meetings. If the vote is almost always unanimous, there is probably strong peer pressure to present a united front or all board members may have similar views. Lack of questions or discussion prior to a vote may also indicate such pressure. Other reasons for a unanimous vote are that board members are not well informed but trust the superintendent's recommendation; or the issue has been discussed between individual members prior to the meeting.

A board member who does not have strong convictions on a particular issue, may vote with the majority to avoid being on the losing side. Many school board members support whatever the administration wants, which brings about the charge that the school board is a "rubber stamp" for the administration. As mentioned earlier, since the board hires the superintendent, they are inclined to trust his or her judgment. Only strong conviction or conflicting evidence would cause board members to oppose the administration.

Even when the entire board does not agree with you, if you can persuade a strong minority to vote your way, then there will be room for negotiating and persuasion. Most boards seem to experience strong peer pressure to cooperate along with a distaste for a split vote. Board members may attend seminars where they are encouraged to work as a "team" with "give and take." One board member said the first training session she attended strongly emphasized that the board not get involved in curriculum development unless it violated policy.

In many cases, if there is a proposal on the agenda, it is likely that it will pass. Both boards and administrators like the vote to be unanimous. If it looks like there will be a split vote, an item may be removed from the agenda to allow more time to work out the problem. In such a situation, the board may depend on the professional judgment of the superintendent and staff, so it will be important to influence these people, if at all possible.

Your state may have an open meetings law forbidding a quorum of board members to meet privately to negotiate, but any number less than a quorum can meet. Administrators may privately address the opposing board members' reservations and board members may lobby each other on certain issues.

G. INFLUENCING THE SCHOOL BOARD

The best way to influence school administrators and board members is to get to know them as individuals. As you learn more about their concerns and beliefs, you will be better prepared to persuade them. You can do this by attending board meetings, through phone calls, letters, lunches or meetings, and providing information that supports your position. You can request a meeting with any number of board members that is less than a quorum if a quorum requires a public meeting including public notification. For example, you could request a meeting with three members of a seven-member board.

Whether in writing or in person, appeal to reason and logic, asking board members to consider what is best for students. Ask board members to express their views and then respond thoughtfully to their questions and reservations. Use credible sources (i.e., tapes, newspaper articles, other school district's policies, videos, research papers, books, etc.) as a basis for your position. Christian sources can be used, but you should attempt to balance them with secular sources. Provide information in small amounts. Too much at one time may result in it being set aside and not read.

If you want a letter to be read by an individual board member only, mark it personal and send it to his or her home or work address. Some districts open all correspondence to school board members.

H. HOW TO BRING THE ISSUE BEFORE A BOARD MEETING

If the superintendent or staff recommend your policy proposal to the board, you can almost be assured that the majority of the board will vote for it. As stated earlier, the board usually trusts the administration and is likely to adopt its recommendations. The administration can bring the proposal to the board by placing it on the agenda.If your efforts fail at the administrative level, it will be necessary to bring the issue to the board yourself. Since board meetings are open to the public and covered by the local press, bringing the issue to the board will cause your efforts to become public if that has not happened previously.

It is best if the administration agrees to place a policy proposal on the school board agenda. However, there are three ways to bring the issue before the board for a vote:

1. In most districts, if two board members support your proposal, they can ask that it be placed on the agenda. Or:

2. You may request in writing that the issue or proposed policy be placed on the next school board agenda. This action on your part could result in a request from administrators for a meeting to discuss the issue, or it could result in an outright rejection.

   If your request is rejected, and the administration makes no attempt to discuss your proposal:

3. Address the school board in a regularly scheduled meeting during the "citizens to be heard" forum. Ask the board to consider your recommendations for a policy.

In any case, notify the media through a press release the day of, or the day prior to the school board meeting. Once the effort becomes public, implement your strategy to use the media to keep attention focused on the issue. (See chapter 8, "Work With the Media.")

If the board does not respond to public pressure, it will be clear that new school board members must be elected to bring about a change. A request for a new policy can now become an election issue. If you anticipate this eventuality, it may be wise to work quietly to persuade the administration and board members until 3-4 months prior to the next school board election. (See chapter 13, "School Board Elections.")

I. ADDRESSING THE SCHOOL BOARD

Citizens may address the school board by signing in just prior to the meeting. Indicate the issue that you want to address by indicating the agenda item number on the sign-in sheet. If you want to bring a concern to the board that is not on the agenda, you should indicate "Citizens To Be Heard," or the name given to the time allotted for that purpose. Time limits may exist, usually of three to five minutes.

The board may vote or take action only on agenda items. They may ask questions or make comments, but not take action on any issue not on the agenda. Law requires the agenda to be publicly posted prior to a meeting, usually 48 hours in advance.

1. What To Do If You Think the Board Supports You

It is likely that the board members have already made up their minds concerning controversial agenda items before they arrive at the meeting. They will probably know how the majority plans to vote. If you know that they are planning to vote your way, you have five goals:

a. to politely reinforce their position and yours;
b. to refute any points the opposition makes;
c. to show your strength;
d. to communicate facts about your position to the public through the media covering the hearing;
e. to persuade any teachers and other staff, or at least cause them to doubt their reason for opposition.

For advice on giving a talk, review Appendices M, N, O and P.

Appendix M
Give a Talk Before an Audience

Appendix N
Useful Verses to Review Before Speaking

Appendix O
Outline of a Sample Talk

Appendix P
Common Arguments and How to Answer Them

2. What To Do If You Think the Board Opposes You

If your proposal is placed on the agenda and you learn that the majority plan to reject it, try to speak with them privately before the meeting. You may be able to convince them to at least table your proposal for more study and information, or to allow time for public response. If there isn't time to reach board members beforehand, or you know they will be against you, you can still gain some ground through your presentation. Here are some goals:

a. communicate your position clearly, with facts;
b. politely refute the opposition;
c. demonstrate the strength of your position with a large turnout in your favor;

d. communicate to the public and media that there is strong support with reasonable justification for your proposal. Note: This advice is also applicable when you are opposing an objectionable program or policy which the board is considering.

You may be unlikely to change minds, but through asking thoughtful questions, you may cause board members to examine their position. This may accomplish two things: Board members may become confused and decide they do not know enough to vote on the issue; or, you may show to the public that the board does not understand the real issues involved. Make sure you have a good idea how a question will be answered before you ask it. Your questions should draw them to your position. If you can expose something significant that they haven't thought of or they can't answer, you will have gained some ground.

Arrange for several people to speak on behalf of the proposal. Meet in advance to discuss what each person will say so that each speaker will develop a different aspect of the issue. Avoid repetition! One or two individuals should sign in to speak last. They should make notes as they listen to other speakers and be prepared to address unanswered questions, rebut the opposition and summarize the appeal for action.

Each speaker should have a double-spaced typewritten statement that can be given to the school board and media representatives. The statement can be read or key points can be addressed by the speaker. Speakers should be prepared to answer questions and they should have supporting documentation. Statements can be prepared for those willing to speak but not able to prepare their own statements.

Speakers should stick to the issue at hand, and the facts presented should focus on your school district. Avoid mentioning inappropriate incidents, books or materials or procedures which pertain to other districts.

Here are appropriate subjects which can be assigned to your speakers:

1. The failure of the contraceptive approach (assuming that your district has or is considering contraceptive instruction);
2. The myth of value-free sex education, the damage from years of so-called value-neutral sex education, the importance of values and clear standards;
3. The need for a policy, states which require the teaching of abstinence;
4. Health issues: contraceptive failure statistics, health problems from promiscuity.

Be sure to study the common myths about abstinence education in Section V. B. of *Has Sex Education Failed Our Teenagers?* Also review the information in Appendices M, N, and O on how to give a talk.

11

IF YOU WIN, FOLLOW THROUGH

If you have won the battle of getting a good policy adopted, then you will want to make sure that it is implemented correctly. Perhaps the board adopted a policy, but guidelines do not yet exist. Perhaps the policy did not go as far as you would have liked. There is still work to be done. The policy needs to be reinforced and monitored. Potential problem areas need to be watched.

A. REINFORCING THE POLICY

Once the policy is adopted you should be alert to efforts to undermine or overturn it. Endeavor to reinforce the policy by demonstrating strong community support.

One of the most important and effective ways to do this is with letters of appreciation to the superintendent and the school board. Letters to the editors of local newspapers are important, too. Letters from professionals such as doctors, nurses, counselors, as well as elected officials have added significance. Encourage letters of support as long as three or four months following the adoption of the policy.

Other helpful actions include:

1. Make supportive comments in interviews, on open-line talk shows, at P.T.A. meetings, and at any other forum.
2. Write an article supporting abstinence education and commending the district for leadership in adopting the policy. Submit the article to local papers.
3. Respond to unfavorable letters to the editor.
4. Monitor the board meetings and respond immediately to any attacks on the policy.

B. MONITORING POLICY IMPLEMENTATION

Once a policy is adopted, its implementation must be overseen. The policy may require that certain materials and programs be eliminated or modified. The district staff's interpretation may be different from yours and or that of the school board. Specific guidelines should be developed for policy implementation and selection of materials. Once the policy is in place, there must be monitoring to assure that programs and materials meet its standards. Parents should be ready to challenge materials which are not in line with the policy.

C. SEX EDUCATION COMMITTEE

One way to address implementation and monitoring is to request that the district select a committee representing the community to review new materials in light of the boards policy. Since the board adopted the policy, they should appoint the committee. There is a risk in that people opposed to the policy could be selected for the committee. Ask the board to consider the following selection criteria:

1. The committee should include:
    a. only those in agreement with the policy (Once a policy has been adopted, it is self-defeating to include those who oppose it in the group assigned to supervise its implementation.);
    b. parents of children currently enrolled in the district;
    c. teachers;
    d. health care professionals;
    e. some of those who worked for the adoption of the policy.
2. The district staff should advise but not be an official part of the committee;
3. All materials must be approved by a majority of the committee, and if there is strong disagreement, the board would decide the matter.

D. HANDLING COMPLAINTS AND PROBLEM AREAS

Parents invariably find it hard to bring their objections to the attention of the schools. Usually there is fear that their child will be embarrassed or treated differently if they complain. The child may beg parents to not say anything, resulting in parents keeping quiet about their concerns. In such a case the school has effectively become a wedge between the parent and child.

Sometimes when parents discuss their concerns with the teacher, the teacher's response is not cooperative. The parent is told, "You're the only one who has ever complained about this." The parental concern never goes any further so the principal and the district administration remain unaware of any problem. When someone finally does breach the levels of intimidation, the administrators may dismiss the complaint, feeling that if there were a real problem, they would have heard about it before now.

Appendix Q
Complaint Inquiry

Concerns about objectionable materials or programs can be handled individually or through your group. If the matter concerns only one child, the parent should handle the matter. However, if the concern has a far-reaching effect, other parents should be involved. In either case, the parent should never go alone to a meeting to discuss a concern. The parent's spouse or a friend should go along. See Appendix Q for specific helps in making an inquiry about concerns.

One way to handle issues of concern is through your group. An issue which has the strength of a group behind it may receive more serious consideration than one raised by an individual. The charge that "you're the only one" certainly will not be valid.

However, many parents are still reluctant to have a group raise an issue on their behalf. They may still feel they and their child are vulnerable to become classified as trouble-makers. One way to handle this is to have your group develop an inquiry procedure that parents can use. This allows the parent to remain anonymous and protects the child. At the same time, the concern is brought to the attention of the district.

When a parent brings a concern to your group, the group can send a letter and a form asking the school personnel to look into the matter. Such an inquiry should not accuse anyone, but merely state the facts concerning the matter. Include any documentation you have such as a student worksheet, assignment instructions, name of film, etc. (See Appendix Q for sample inquiry form and cover letter.)

For example, a student refused to complete a survey which had been developed by another student; instead she gave it to her parents. The survey included questions such as, "Are you sexually active? Do you take precautions? What kind?" The parents gave the survey to their local chapter of Citizens for Excellence in Education. CEE sent an inquiry (using the form in Appendix Q) to the district office. The form was not returned, but the principal of the high school involved responded by letter. He explained the survey was developed by a student as a result of an English assignment. The students were required to write a persuasive term paper which was to be defended by data supported by a survey or questionnaire.

The principal stated, "In evaluating the questionnaire, there is question as to the suitability of the topic for an English class, but not a question as to the assignment." He added that he had spoken with the teacher and "advised her to be more selective in the subject matter approved for an English term paper." The inquiry gained a responsive explanation with no embarrassment for the student or parents. The principal and teacher know that parents are concerned about this type of assignment. This teacher is likely to be more careful in the future, and the word will probably spread to other teachers.

The nature of your inquiry and the response of school personnel can be printed in your newsletter to inform other parents. If the district refuses to respond, you can forward the matter to the school board. If necessary, you can raise the issue at a public board meeting and disseminate to the press information about the issue and the lack of response by the district to parental concerns. In other words, you can continually push for accountability.

Copies of the inquiry and the results should be maintained in a file. They can be used if needed to demonstrate an on-going problem.

E. A FINAL AREA OF CONCERN: YOUR STATE

Even though you may achieve success in your district, it is essential that you become informed about what is happening at the state level. All of your efforts could be undone or undermined by legislation or a state board ruling. In the same way you became concerned about the values your school board members hold, you need to be concerned about your state school officials and your state legislators.

For example, since 1987, Planned Parenthood, a national organization which receives millions of our tax dollars, has listed seven states (Connecticut, Nevada, Oregon, Texas, Vermont, Virginia and Wisconsin) in their "Tier I" category to push for state-mandated comprehensive sex education. Ten other states are listed as Tier II targets and the rest are in Tier III.

For several years in Texas, Planned Parenthood has worked hand-in-hand with a large school district and the state education agency. The state agency wrote a curriculum, Planned Parenthood used their resources to promote it and train teachers, and it was piloted in that district. The state education agency held a state-wide conference for educators to unveil and promote the new curriculum, and the agency allowed Planned Parenthood to help promote it. Legislation was introduced in 1987 that would have mandated use of that curriculum. Two legislators were invited to the state conference to promote their bills. The legislation was defeated, largely due to groups of parents across the state who expressed their opposition. However, the state agency continues to promote the curriculum across the state at regional training workshops and the state school board conventions.

Again in 1989, bills were introduced that would mandate comprehensive sex education. At the same time, legislation requiring abstinence instruction whenever sex education is taught was stonewalled by one committee head who refused to let the bill be heard.

The amount of time and effort that have been devoted to mandate comprehensive sex education at state levels is an indication of the resources and dedication of those behind the effort. They have solicited the support of major organizations, such as the P.T.A., even though the rank and file P.T.A. membership has no idea of the content of the curriculum.

It is clear that we must remain alert. We are in an intense struggle for the minds and hearts of our children, and far too many parents seem unaware of the danger. Organizations which monitor legislation and can help you to keep informed include Concerned Women of America and Eagle Forum. See Appendix Y for addresses.

Appendix Y
National Organizations that Have Local Chapters

12

IF YOU LOSE, THEN WHAT?

"Never tire of doing what is right!"

2 Thessalonians 3:13

If you did not accomplish the goal you had hoped to achieve, you might be tempted to feel defeated. You will need to put all that has happened in perspective. Here are some things you may have accomplished:

- Parents in the district have become more aware and concerned about their schools.
- Because you spoke out, other parents gained confidence to speak out.
- There is more accountability on the part of the district because you have surfaced concerns. You can be sure that decision-makers will be concerned about your reaction to any new materials or programs.
- Your position has gained credibility.
- You have laid the foundation for future efforts.

A defeat can sometimes mobilize the community. Those who sat by while your group worked may now realize they need to be involved. They may have felt secure that you were working for what they believed; the loss may shock them into action.

Besides seeing the good results that occurred as a result of your efforts, keep your group mobilized in order to more fully achieve your desired ends.

A. WORK TO ELECT BOARD MEMBERS WHO REPRESENT YOUR VIEWS

Since the school board is the key to policy changes, continue working toward electing board members who share your concerns and who are willing to initiate changes. See chapter 13, School Board Elections.

B. KEEP UP PUBLIC PRESSURE

Perseverance can be a key to victory.

In Luke 18, Jesus told his disciples a parable about an unjust judge who neither feared God nor respected men. At first he refused the pleas of a widow asking for justice. Yet, because of her persistence, he granted her request. Like the widow, you will need to communicate to the district that you and those who share your views are not going away; you will be there to call them to accountability.

You can keep up the pressure by letters to the editor and other media efforts, petition efforts, monitoring and speaking at board meetings, and keeping parents informed through a newsletter. Press releases can be issued to commend positive action and object to inappropriate action. Ask local radio talk shows to have guests who can discuss the issues. Provide them with information on suggested speakers. Repetition as well as new perspectives are important.

C. COUNTER NEGATIVE TEACHING

If you are unsuccessful in having objectionable material removed from the classroom, then you will need to counter the teaching being given in the schools whether or not your children are exempted from attending sex education classes. Use some of the resources listed in the appendices of the sex education report and this handbook in order to know which books, tapes, etc. to purchase for the training of your own children.

D. EXCUSE YOUR CHILD FROM OBJECTIONABLE SEX EDUCATION

If your child is scheduled for a sex education program, attend the parents' presentation. Ask for an outline of materials and any handouts. See any films or videos and ask about how various questions will be answered. This will help you to decide if you want your child to participate.

At the elementary level, most schools actively recruit parental participation and permission. Take advantage of this opportunity to examine the materials and discuss them with your child prior to the classroom presentation. Failure to do this will rob you of the opportunity to be the first person to explain these sensitive matters to your child. What you do at this point will set the stage for future discussions.

It is also our opinion that at the elementary level, parents should not allow their children to be part of the class presentation. The parent can share the content with the child and explain that it is a special subject which deserves the privacy of personal discussion at home. Tell the child that there are certain matters which are not appropriate for group discussion, especially since the school is not likely to have a biblical perspective which reflects your family's values.

At the middle school level (junior high), the school may attempt to notify parents, but not require permission. It is best to call the school or district office soon after the beginning of the school year to determine what will be taught and when.

At the high school level, there may be no attempt to notify parents, and parents will have to dig for the information. Some parents discovered that students in a Child Development class receive a graphic contraceptive presentation. Never in their wildest imagination would they have thought that contraceptives had a place in "child development."

If you decide you do not want your child in a presentation, most schools will allow you to exempt him or her. This is commonly referred to as "opting out." The child does not go with the class to the presentation, or leaves the classroom prior to the presentation. Usually, this sets the child apart from the others, risking ridicule from the rest of the students. A wedge is driven between parent and child if the child resents "being treated like a baby" or views mom and dad as prudes.

A parent who anticipates this reaction may decide the presentation is "not that bad," and will allow the child to attend. However, if something is "not that bad," then it is "not that good" either. As parents, we should strive for the best.

One way around the standard procedure of opting out is to arrange a legitimate excused absence for your child on the date of the presentation. Schedule an eye or ear exam, a dental or medical appointment. A little known fact is that most schools allow a student to be released for religious purposes. Using this right, one or more parents can schedule an appointment when their pastor can talk with their children about a biblical perspective on marriage and family. The pastor can explain to the children that sex education belongs at home and in the church, then explain the Bible's view of love and marriage. At the middle school or high school level, a group program may be offered by the pastor or youth leader during the time the school has their instruction.

Parents need to take the leadership and find creative ways to counteract a negative program at school. Be prepared before decisions are made for you.

E. SET UP A LENDING LIBRARY AND SPEAKERS BUREAU

If you purchased sample curricula and audiovisual resources in order to show to school personnel, you could now make those items available to teachers who would like to use them in the classroom. Even though you might not have been able to get the entire school board to support your proposal, you probably met some supportive teachers who favor the teaching of abstinence. Keep a good relationship with the supportive teachers, and let them borrow your resources.

Besides lending out your materials, consider forming a speakers bureau for your organization. Gather resources (i.e. some of the items listed in the appendices of this manual), develop some talks, prepare a list of your materials, notify teachers, and be available to give presentations in the classroom. Speakers bureaus are an effective means for getting the abstinence message to students.

F. HOLD COMMUNITY BASED ABSTINENCE EDUCATION PROGRAMS

Get a group of churches or organizations to sponsor a "Why Wait?" conference in your community. Bring in a qualified and effective speaker to talk to teens, to parents, and to pastors. Obtain the Josh McDowell *Why Wait? Action Packet* for more information. Refer to Appendix AA.

Appendix AA
Books to Guide Parents

G. HOLD TEACHER TRAINING CONFERENCES

In many communities, one of the ways to bring about an awareness of the importance and effectiveness of abstinence education is to bring in a teacher trainer from one of the national organizations (i.e., Project Respect, Teen-Aid, Respect, Inc.). Check with your state's central education agency to find out the necessary steps to follow in order for conference attendees to receive advanced academic credit.

Promote the conference with mailouts, newspaper and radio announcements, newsletters, etc. Stress the credit points to be given to teachers who attend.

Conferences such as this can help to convince school personnel that abstinence education is the right approach for the school. Eventually, the school district might become more favorable to adopting an abstinence policy that will assure that the school district upholds a high standard.

13

SCHOOL BOARD ELECTIONS

Since the school board is the key to policy change, it is important to assure that board members represent you. If you were unable to accomplish your goal because of resistance from the board, then it's time to get a new board!

Non-profit organizations are not allowed by law to endorse candidates. They can, however, provide information to candidates, hold candidates forums, and conduct candidate surveys. A separate group or election committee should be established to select and support school board candidates.

School board elections are usually non-partisan. A typical school board has 7 positions with a 3-year term of office. Ideally, the terms of office are staggered so that not all positions are up for election at the same time.

In some districts, school boards are carefully controlled by the current board or administrators. Candidates will be selected unofficially and quietly behind the scenes. Then the board and administrators will endorse those candidates publicly.

A board member who does not plan to run for reelection might resign early in order for the board to appoint a replacement. The outsider is put in the position of running against an incumbent.

The board may elect as its officers those whose term of office expires that year. The outsider is faced with not only running against an incumbent, but against an officer of the board.

The district administration can cooperate by giving incumbent candidates as much publicity and other help as possible. They will be the speakers at dedications, graduations, awards ceremonies and P.T.A. meetings. Their campaign literature will be placed in teachers' mailboxes. They will be given the opportunity to lead school tours.

A. ORGANIZE A CANDIDATE SELECTION COMMITTEE

A candidate selection committee acts somewhat like a nominating committee. It should include trusted individuals who will meet to discuss the selection of candidates, question potential candidates, select candidates, and to work to get candidates elected. A chairman of the committee should be appointed, and the committee should meet regularly to work toward the goal of the election of the candidates. The committee should also develop a platform on the issues.

B. GUIDELINES FOR SELECTION OF CANDIDATES

These guidelines are intended to be used in considering the selection of a candidate. No one person can be the perfect candidate. However, the potential candidate must share your values, be willing to learn, and be willing to run for office.

1. Electability
   - a. Name recognition, or ability to get name recognition prior to the election. Factors to consider are:
     1. Previous candidacy for public office
     2. Positive media exposure
   - b. Potential to gain endorsements
   - c. Reputation in the community
     1. How is the potential candidate perceived in the community
     2. Honest, good character
   - d. Public speaking ability: good vocabulary and presentation; articulate

2. Positive Indicators
   - a. Children attending, or graduated, from public school
   - b. Time available for public speaking and campaigning
   - c. Commitment to study the issues, to devoting time necessary
   - d. Ability to raise funds (known among people willing to contribute)
   - e. Compatibility to current sympathetic board members or other candidates your committee will support

3. Knowledge and Position on the Issues
   - a. Ability to discuss issues, identify problem areas, and recommend solutions
   - b. Knowledge of a range of education issues of concern in the district
   - c. Strong stand on key issues and willingness to speak out
   - d. Willing to stand alone, initiate action, question an issue

C. DEVELOP AND USE A CANDIDATE SCREENING SURVEY

Use a candidate screening survey during the selection process in order to provide information about potential candidates to the candidate selection committee. A screening survey will help you to know if the interested persons agree with your platform. When developing a survey, consider what information might be helpful to your committee in selecting a candidate. Include issues of concern in your district.

Ideally, there should be a variety of individuals who are willing and ready to run for school board. Encourage those who think they might be interested in being a candidate to complete a survey. During the selection process, some individuals might realize they are not prepared to run. Their involvement can prepare them to run in the future. Or, they may discover their talents and resources can be used in other ways, such as lobbying the board, writing letters, raising money, etc. Being a part of the process can be a valuable experience.

Ask each potential candidate to respond in writing to the screening survey. Or, potential candidates can be asked to respond verbally to the questions in a candidate selection committee meeting.

Perhaps your committee has only been able to select one candidate who is willing to run and there are two or three board positions open. Others, who you don't know may have heard that you are backing candidates, may contact you, or someone's name may have been recommended to you. You can use the screening survey to gather initial information about these individuals.

The information in the screening survey can be helpful when you are enlisting support for your candidates among your friends who may not know them. The information can also help you to know in which areas your candidate needs to be more informed.

Appendix V contains a sample cover letter, candidate survey, and screening form that can be used in assessing the qualifications and views of candidates.

Appendix V
Sample School Board Candidate Screening Forms

D. HOST A "MEET THE CANDIDATES NIGHT"

Although other groups, such as teachers' unions or P.T.A.s may hold a candidates forum, they usually do not deal adequately with the issues of concern to Christian parents. Having a candidates' night can help to make the Christian community aware of the school board election and the issues. A candidates' forum can awaken the Christian community to the school board election and the issues, and it can build momentum for the candidates.

Here are some guidelines:

1. Set a date (after the filing deadline) and notify all candidates at least one week in advance. Be sure the date does not conflict with regularly scheduled board meetings, other candidate forums or major events which could reduce attendance.

2. Recruit a committee to sponsor the candidates' night. If a member of your group is running for school board, then it would be best to recruit another group or individuals who are not a part of your group as the hosts. Some churches may be willing to host the event.

3. Publicize the event through public service announcements on radio, newsletters and fliers which you can distribute at local churches and other sites.

4. Plan a format and select a moderator. Each candidate should have a timed period to speak (3-5 minutes) and be asked questions from a panel and the audience.

5. Invite candidates to bring their election literature and signs.

One church has hosted a candidates' night for several years. The candidates have been invited to give their position on several issues in two or three minutes. At first, that seemed impossible to do, yet it turned out to be quite easy and helpful to summarize the central issues of the election. Following the candidates' statements, they were questioned by a panel and then by the audience. The candidate surveys were also distributed, helping the audience identify areas in which the candidates differed.

E. SUGGESTIONS TO HELP ELECT CANDIDATES

1. Join local organizations (i.e., homeowners and taxpayers associations) that have goals with which you agree. Ask them to inform their membership of your candidacy.
2. Arrange for a commercial on your local Christian radio station. The commercial should run for a least five days.
3. Write letters to the editors of daily and weekly newspapers. (See sample.)
4. Obtain voters lists from last year's school board election. Underline those known by campaign workers. Place their names on a list to call and request support. (Since few vote in school board elections, those who voted last year are likely to vote again.)
5. Plan candidate literature and signs.
6. Request endorsements and use on campaign literature.
7. Sign up campaign workers and poll workers.
8. Organize a phone bank. Obtain lists of names from groups and friends. The day before the election, call to remind people to vote and ask for support.
9. Take advantage of "open-lines" on talk radio by having your supporters call in.
10. Contact your party precinct chairmen. You can get their names by contacting party headquarters.
11. Do not consider endorsements from teachers associations that are affiliated with the National Education Association (NEA), or other organizations which have goals in conflict with yours.
12. Hold candidate coffees and fundraisers where people can meet the candidate.
13. Ask friends to write letters, mail campaign literature, and contact their friends.
14. Try to enlist help from veteran campaign workers.
15. Issue press releases to make the candidate's position known.

14

CONCLUSION

"No one else dared join them;
even though they were highly regarded by the people."

Acts 5:13

Most of us are not in a position to make changes in teachers' colleges, teachers' unions, or in curriculum development. Others will have to see this need and decide to work in these crucial areas. Still, we wield significant influence at the local and the state level through our input as citizens and our involvement in the election process. The responsibility for positive changes ultimately lies with local school boards, parents, and other concerned citizens. We can be "wall-builders" as the people were in Nehemiah's time.

Sooner or later anyone in a leadership position will receive admiration. Admiration is nice (if you're a statue or a work of art), but it doesn't accomplish anything. Most of us do not need admiration. We need encouragement, prayers, and if possible, active help. Sometimes admiration can even be a source of discouragement. We are told, "I really admire what you are doing, but I could never do it," or "I'm not called to do that, I don't have any patience." On the other hand, one man was a real source of encouragement when he said, "It really blesses my heart to know what you're doing; we're praying for you."

As writers of this manual, we ask, "Don't admire us. Join us!" As leaders in your schools and community, you need to say the same to those you contact: "Don't admire us. Join us!"

We hope that this manual has been a source of help and encouragement to you. We trust that you will use what you have learned to train and encourage others. Finally, we desire that you will pray that the Lord will raise up leaders in other areas to help restore the values upon which our nation was founded.

Appendices

A. Set Up a Prayer Network 79
B. Differing Views: What People Think of Each Other 81
C. Tips for Gathering Information by Phone 85
D. The Teenage Sexuality Crisis in the Community 87
E. Programs for Teens in the Community 89
F. The State's Education Structure 90
G. State Laws About Sex Education 92
H. Locating Information in the District 93
I. School District Information 94
J. The School's Sex Education Program 95
K. Abstinence Programs Elsewhere in Your Region 98
L. Evaluating Your School's Sex Education Program 99
M. Giving a Talk Before an Audience 101
N. Useful Verses to Review Before Speaking 108
O. Outline of a Sample Talk 111
P. Common Arguments and How to Answer Them 113
Q. Complaint Inquiry 115
R. Specific Helps for Parents and Guiding Principles 118
S. Sample Petition 121
T. Sample Letters to the Editor 123
U. Sample Press Releases 126
V. Sample School Board Candidate Screening Forms 128
W. Publishers of Abstinence Education Materials 131
X. Periodicals that Cover Education Issues 133
Y. National Organizations that Have Local Chapters 134
Z. Glossary of Terms 135
AA. Books to Guide Parents 139
BB. Audiovisual Resources for Adults on Teenage Sexuality 141
CC. Books for Teens 143
DD. Tapes for Teens 144
EE. Books to Help Parents Teach Children 145
FF. Tapes to Help Parents Teach Children 146
GG. Pamphlets to Help Parents Teach Children 147

APPENDIX

A

Set Up a Prayer Network

1. Find a person who will volunteer to coordinate a prayer network.
2. Prepare a list of specific prayer needs. Put the prayer requests on a sheet so that everyone can pray specifically. See the sample prayer request sheet below.
3. Hold prayer meetings at regular intervals and before important meetings with school officials.
4. Set up a telephone prayer chain so that people can pray at specific times.
5. Keep people updated on the answers to prayer.

SAMPLE PRAYER REQUEST SHEET

NATION

1. That there will be a spiritual awakening in this country
2. That God's people will humble themselves and pray
3. That those in leadership will seek righteousness

FAMILIES

1. That there will be godly leadership in the home
2. That there will be love between parents
3. That there will be love for children
4. That there will be biblical guidance for children

TEENAGERS

1. That teenagers will find salvation and lordship in Jesus Christ
2. That teenagers will obey God's commandments, particularly in the area of sexual conduct
3. That teenagers will have the strength to resist negative influences
4. That Christian teenagers will set a positive example in their schools

SCHOOL DECISION-MAKERS

1. That school decision makers will realize the need to uphold positive principles as embodied in our Judeo-Christian heritage
2. That school leaders will have wisdom in making decisions
3. That school leaders will select the right policies, guidelines, and materials for students

PARENT-SCHOOL INTERACTION

1. That Christian parents who interact with the schools will rely on God's strength
2. That Christian parents will be blameless before God for their conduct
3. That Christian parents will have wisdom in their conversations with school officials
4. That school leaders will be receptive to godly input
5. That the pure motives of Christian parents will not be maligned

SPECIFICS

1. Names of Christian parents who are undertaking the task of interacting with the schools:
   ____
2. Time and dates to pray for them:____________________________
3. People with whom they will interact:__________________________
4. The specific purpose of the interaction:________________________

APPENDIX

B

Differing Views: What People Think of Each Other

A major metropolitan newspaper ran a front page story concerning sex education in the local schools. One of the people embroiled in the conflict was quoted: "It's part of a network of extremist groups moving insidiously to impose its values on America's children. The impact of their power is that the health of our children has been placed in jeopardy. We don't see their approach as inclusive and we don't see that as appropriate."

After reading the quotation, one might assume that the person was concerned about some bizarre group trying to impose radical views on the children in the community. Surprisingly though, the person was referring to a group of parents headed by Anne Newman, one of the authors of this *Parents' Handbook*. The person also made critical remarks at a committee meeting about Dinah Richard, the other author of this handbook.

Just think—two homemakers, who faithfully cook meals for their families, drive carpools, attend church regularly, cook brownies for fundraisers, and who are otherwise no threat to the world, suddenly become "dangerous" when they begin to express concern about what is being taught in the classroom.

We should not be too surprised to discover that this type of reaction occurs. There is that famous adage "Never discuss sex, religion, or politics." Sex education, more than any other subject, includes all three of those ingredients.

Before you begin to interact with your school officials regarding sex education, it would be helpful to realize the different perspectives people have. By realizing the different views, you might be able to develop a better strategy that will reduce these preconceived notions and allow you to proceed with a rational discussion of the issue of sex education.

How Do School Officials View Themselves?

Most school personnel are caring professionals who are often overworked, underpaid, and unappreciated. Any person who has been in the school system very long will confirm this. They will also tell you that they get blamed for every evil that befalls society. They are treated disrespectfully by students and others.

Considering the years of education they acquired and the on-going training they must obtain, school personnel understandably feel that their professionalism is being questioned when parents disagree with what is being taught in the school.

While parents might feel intimidated when some school personnel become defensive about inquiries, parents must not assume that a workable solution cannot be achieved. Instead, parents need to view school officials as their allies, not their enemies. Many school officials are loving, caring parents just like you.

There are, however, some school personnel whom you will not be able to reach. One type is the school official who has become the "surrogate parent," believing that parents don't care about their children, that parents are ill-equipped to educate their children about sex education, and that parents are willing to transfer their roles over to the schools in the area of sex education. While it is true that school officials encounter some parents who fit these categories, it is wrong for school officials to paint all parents with that brush. Ironically, while complaining about lack of parental concern, this type of school official does not welcome parental input concerning sex education if the parents' views do not coincide with his or hers.

A second type of school official to be concerned about is the "change agent." This type of person goes beyond the simple "surrogate parent" and believes that traditional Judeo-Christian morality is dangerous, that children need to be liberated from their parents' views, and that children's rights are more important than parents' rights. Fortunately, the "change agent" is rare in the local school district, but the presence of one is often very powerful.

How Do School Officials View Christian Parents Who Complain About Sex Education?

Earlier, you read an excerpt from a newspaper in which a person labeled concerned Christian parents as "extremists." Unfortunately, that is usually the portrayal in the media. Thus, it is understandable why school personnel and others in the community may adopt a similar view toward caring parents. But even without local media coverage of your interaction with the schools, you need to anticipate that some school personnel will have the following preconceived views toward you.

1. The intellect of parents: the belief that parents are narrow-minded, they are not inclusive, and they are uneducated about the subject. (The assumption is that the school official is broad-minded, inclusive, and educated.)
2. The stability of parents: the belief that the parents are irrational, emotional, and volatile. (Conversely, the school official is rational, non-emotional, and stable.)
3. The foundation of the parents' views: the belief that the parents have no scientific basis for their views, they are naively idealistic, and they are not contemporary. (Conversely, the school personnel are scientific, pragmatic, and modern.)

4. The religious beliefs of parents: the belief that the parents are religious zealots, self-righteous, and are secretly trying to get the Bible taught in school. (Conversely, the school official is moderate, humble, and doesn't have a hidden agenda.)
5. The parents' association with a national conspiracy: the belief that the parents are part of a national right-wing movement, they are trying to take over the schools, they are trying to censor books, and they are a vocal minority. (Conversely, the school official is moderate, is trying to work within the system, favors openness, and is representative of the mainstream.)
6. The ability of parents to cooperate with the school: the belief that the parents are troublemakers, they can't get along with school officials, and they are impeding progress. (Conversely, school officials are helpers, they try to cooperate, and they are facilitating progress.)

How Do Christian Parents View the Schools?

Often parents assume that if school personnel are unresponsive to their views, then that means that the school officials are wicked. A more accurate view should be that most school personnel are unaware of the harm that is being done by teaching the wrong approach. Some school officials place their trust in groups that promote contraceptive based sex education. Some are misled to believe that the teaching of morality is the same as religious indoctrination. Some school administrators are unaware of what is being taught in the classroom. Some are misinformed about their state's policies. Others are forced to teach the wrong approach. Some have tried to get good programs, but they represent the minority, and, therefore, they are intimidated into silence. Some have their hands tied.

Regardless of what the school officials believe, parents need to treat them respectfully. Parents should recognize the advantages of a school system and work within it to achieve change. Moreover, God admonishes us to pray for those in authority and to be obedient to the laws.

How Do Christian Parents View Themselves?

Some parents often develop a feeling of inadequacy toward themselves if they don't hold an academic degree. Sometimes they are intimidated by the credentials and titles of educators.

Sometimes that feeling of inadequacy carries over into questioning the basis of their own views. However, feelings of doubt do not have to be a negative experience. Uncertainty can lead to deep introspection about your views, the basis for your views, and the outward manner in which you express your views. Proper alignment with God and pure motives is what is most important.

Sometimes when a parent is told that he or she is the only one who has complained about the school's sex education program (which is a frequent remark used by school personnel), it leads the parent to feel isolated. Then when people begin to ridicule the parent, the parent in turn might feel persecuted. While it is true that the world will not love you, the parent needs to get rid of the martyr complex and develop a positive self-image.

Assess the things that are in your favor. If you are presenting a truthful message, then the truth is on your side. If you are presenting your views in a loving manner, then you will be pleasing to God. If you are presenting facts, then science is on your side. If your family agrees with what you are doing, then you have the favor of your family. And even if you don't hear from others in your community, you must realize that there are many parents who admire what you are doing.

You have many sound reasons to nourish a positive image of what you are trying to accomplish in your community.

APPENDIX

C

Tips for Gathering Information by Phone

1. Use the telephone directory or school directory to find out the correct office and phone number to call. If you are uncertain, dial the main office.
2. Always have a full sheet of paper in front of you. Before you place the call, list the date and time. When you place your first call, write the number down on your sheet. List the name of the person with whom you speak, i.e., Mrs. Jones, superintendent's office, 555-5535.
3. Open with your name, a simple statement of why you are calling, and a question asking if you have contacted the correct office. If you are not calling the right office, ask which one to call. Then write down that number and office name on your sheet of paper.
4. Dial the new number. Again state your name. Tell who referred you to this number (i.e., "Mrs. Jones in the superintendent's office said that you are the person who can help me"). Repeat your name and why you are calling.
5. You might have to repeat this process several times until you reach the right person who can help you.
6. If the person says it will be necessary to call you back, be sure to ask when you should expect the call. Make a note of that on your sheet. Give the person adequate time to return your call. If the person has not returned your call, then call back.
7. Anticipate that when you begin to make inquiries about certain issues over the telephone, the receptionist or secretary might become suspicious about you. Prepare some answers. For example:

   "I am new to this subject and I want to be a conscientious parent."

   "Too many parents are unconcerned. I want to be a good parent and work with the schools."

   "I want to become more active in the schools and I am seeking information from you because you are the best source. I don't want to depend on second-hand information."
8. If the person becomes hostile, use some statements to show that you are not launching a personal attack.

   "No doubt, it's no fun receiving complaints from parents. I can appreciate what you have to go through."

"Thank you for taking time to help me. I know you're very busy and I'm an unplanned interruption."

"I believe it's unfair when people attack a program or policy without thoroughly investigating. I want to make sure I'm not like those people."

"I hope I didn't catch you at a bad moment. Is there a more convenient time I can call you?"

9. Once you reach the right source and you begin to receive the information you are seeking, then take notes as the person is talking. Occasionally, stop the conversation and repeat what you've written down so that the person can verify it for you. Use the forms in Appendices D and E of this manual to record the information.
10. Ask the person if you can obtain copies of the information. If so, find out the correct procedure. Write down the procedure on your paper. Immediately follow the procedure. If the person says that you can come to the office to pick it up, then ask when it would be convenient. If you are referred to another office, then call that office, using the name of the person you talked with as a referral.
11. End all of your calls with a question asking if there are other useful people or sources that you could contact.
12. Express your appreciation. If the person mails you information, drop a return note saying that it arrived. Thank the person again.
13. Keep your telephone notes for future reference in case you need to obtain more information. Your notes might be useful years down the road.

APPENDIX

D

The Teenage Sexuality Crisis in the Community

Attach photocopies of detailed reports if they are available.

TEENAGE POPULATION (Sources of information:____________________)

	Current Year________	Past Year________
# teens in county	________	________
# teens in city	________	________
# teens in middle school	________	________
# teens in high school	________	________

TEENAGE PREGNANCIES (Sources of information:____________________)

	Current Year________	Past Year________
# pregnancies in county	________	________
# pregnancies in city	________	________
# pregnancies in school dist.	________	________

TEENAGE ABORTIONS (Sources of information:____________________)

	Current Year________	Past Year________
# abortions	________	________

TEENAGE BIRTHS (Sources of information:____________________)

	Current Year________	Past Year________
# births to all females in city/county	________	________
# births to teenagers in city/county	________	________
# births to teenagers in school district	________	________

MAKE SEVERAL COPIES BEFORE COMPLETING

SCHOOL DROPOUTS (Sources of information:______________________________)

	Current Year__________	Past Year__________
Total # school dropouts	__________	__________
# dropouts due to pregnancy	__________	__________

SEXUALLY TRANSMITTED DISEASES (Sources:______________________________)

	Current Year__________	Past Year__________
# reported STDs in county	__________	__________
# reported STDs to teenagers	__________	__________

DEMOGRAPHIC DATA ABOUT PREGNANT TEENS

(Sources:______________________________)

Marital status of parents______________________________

Socioeconomic background______________________________

Family conditions______________________________

Drug or alcohol problems______________________________

Academic performance______________________________

Religiosity______________________________

Other:______________________________

OTHER PROBLEMS AFFECTING TEENAGERS

(Sources:______________________________)

MAKE SEVERAL COPIES BEFORE COMPLETING

APPENDIX

E

Programs for Teens in the Community

NAME OF ORGANIZATION________________________________

CONTACT PERSON________________________________

ADDRESS________________________________

CITY________________________ STATE__________ ZIP__________

PHONE________________________________

OBJECTIVE/PURPOSE OF THE ORGANIZATION________________________________

____

AFFILIATION OF THE ORGANIZATION________________________________

BELIEFS OF THE ORGANIZATION________________________________

____

____

DESCRIPTION OF PROGRAM DEALING WITH TEEN SEXUALITY, HEALTH CARE, SERVICES, ETC.________________________________

____

____

DOES THE ORGANIZATION INTERACT WITH SCHOOLS IN THE AREA?__________

IF SO, IN WHAT WAY?________________________________

EFFECTIVENESS OF THE PROGRAM________________________________

____

WILL ORGANIZATION SEND LITERATURE ABOUT THEIR PROGRAM FOR TEENS?______

DOES ORGANIZATION UPHOLD TRADITIONAL VALUES?________________

____

DOES ORGANIZATION USE THE WRONG APPROACHES TO THE ADOLESCENT SEXUALITY CRISIS?________________________________

SPECIFY (contraceptives? abortion? etc.?):________________________________

DOES ORGANIZATION HAVE APPROPRIATE SEX EDUCATION MATERIALS?__________

SPECIFY:________________________________

MAKE SEVERAL COPIES BEFORE COMPLETING

APPENDIX

F

The State's Education Structure

STATE BOARD OF EDUCATION

Address:__________

City:__________

Chairman:__________

Number of Board Members:__________

Board Members:

Name:	Address:	City:	Phone:

1.__________

2.__________

3.__________

4.__________

5.__________

6.__________

7.__________

8.__________

9.__________

10.__________

Are members elected or appointed?__________

Term of Office:__________

When are elections held?__________

Elected by district or at large?__________

State Commissioner or Superintendent of Education:__________

Deputy Commissioner or Superintendent:__________

What statutes govern the State Board and the public education system? (i.e., laws, education code, constitution)__________

MAKE SEVERAL COPIES BEFORE COMPLETING

STATE LEGISLATURE

How many senators:__________ How many representatives:__________

Your state senator:__________

Address__________

Phone__________

Your state representative:__________

Address__________

Phone__________

Senate Education Committee Members:

1.__________	6.__________	11.__________
2.__________	7.__________	12.__________
3.__________	8.__________	13.__________
4.__________	9.__________	14.__________
5.__________	10.__________	15.__________

House Education Committee Members

1.__________	6.__________	11.__________
2.__________	7.__________	12.__________
3.__________	8.__________	13.__________
4.__________	9.__________	14.__________
5.__________	10.__________	15.__________

REGIONAL EDUCATION AGENCIES:

Number of regions:__________

What region are you in?__________

Purpose of regional agency:__________

INDEPENDENT SCHOOL DISTRICTS

Number of districts in state:__________

Your district's rank in size (i.e., 3rd largest).__________

MAKE SEVERAL COPIES BEFORE COMPLETING

APPENDIX

G

State Laws About Sex Education

Does the state mandate:	By Law	Bill #	By Essential Element* (List subject areas)
1. Sex Education?**			
2. Sexually Transmitted Diseases Education?			
3. AIDS Education?			

Is there a state curriculum for:	Mandated? (Indicate title of curriculum)	Optional?
1. Sex education?**		
2. Sexually Transmitted Diseases Education?		
3. AIDS Education?		

Are there state approved audiovisual aids for sex education?______________________________

Where can the list be obtained?______________________________

____

What educational background is required to teach sex education?

____

____

____

What training does the state offer teachers of sex education?

____

____

* Essential Elements are specific concepts that are required in certain subject areas

** Sex Education is sometimes called "family life education" or "human growth and reproduction"

APPENDIX

H

Locating Information in the District

The questions below will aid you in finding items of information that you will find helpful. Some districts may use different terms (i.e., administrative guidelines, regulations, etc.). A school personnel directory may not be available to the public, but an organizational chart of administrators and a listing of school principals may be.

In general, don't ask if there is a charge. Much of the information should be available to the public. Initial copies will probably be provided free of charge. However, when groups become involved, some districts assess a per-page fee to recover costs. Sometimes the fee is out of line in order to discourage parents from obtaining a lot of information. Fees should be comparable to local copying costs. If they are excessive, ask to borrow the materials and copy them yourself.

Where can a school personnel directory be obtained?____________________

____

Where can district policies and guidelines be reviewed?____________________

____

Where can copies be obtained?______________________________

Where can a list of curriculum materials be reviewed and obtained?____________________

____

Does the district have a parental complaint procedure regarding materials and programs?________

____

Where can a copy of the procedure be obtained?____________________

____

What is the procedure for a change in policies and guidelines?____________________

____

____

____

What is the procedure for selection and adoption of curricula?____________________

____

____

For supplemental classroom materials?______________________________

____

MAKE SEVERAL COPIES BEFORE COMPLETING

APPENDIX

I

School District Information

ADMINISTRATIVE INFORMATION

Administrative Staff: (Ask for an organizational chart)

Superintendent____________________

Deputy/Assistant Superintendent____________________

Superintendent of Instruction____________________

Name/Title of Person Responsible For:

Elementary Education____________________

Secondary Education____________________

Health Programs____________________

Science Department____________________

Home Economics Programs____________________

Other administrators____________________

____

____

How many schools in district?__________ How many students?__________

How many elementary schools?__________ How many students?__________

How many middle schools (jr. high)?__________ How many students?__________

How many high schools?__________ How many students?__________

MAKE SEVERAL COPIES BEFORE COMPLETING

APPENDIX

J

The School's Sex Education Program

NAME OF PROGRAM:____

1. **LAW AND POLICY, AND MATERIALS RELATED TO THE PROGRAMS.** Obtain a copy or review the following:

   ______ Laws related to the program

   ______ District's Philosophy of Education statement

   ______ Policies related to the program

   ______ Guidelines related to the program

   ______ Written rationale for program

   ______ Program curriculum or outline

   ______ Supplemental material (films, handouts, reading assignments, etc.)

   ______ List of resources (special speakers, referral agencies, etc.)

   ______ List of courses in which the subject is covered

2. **BACKGROUND OF THE PROGRAM**

   When did the program begin in the district?________________________

   Who developed it?____________________________________

   Have any studies been conducted regarding it?______________________

3. **WHO IS RESPONSIBLE FOR THE PROGRAM**

   Title:____

   Supervisor:_____________________________________

   Qualifications required:______________________________

   Who selects materials:_______________________________

   Who approves materials:______________________________

   Who conducts instruction (teacher/nurse/counselor/other):

   ____

MAKE SEVERAL COPIES BEFORE COMPLETING

Was the program adopted by the school board?__________

Were materials reviewed and approved by the school board?__________

Who selects outside speakers/groups to be invited into the schools?

____

4. COMPLAINT PROCEDURE

Ask for a copy of the complaint/grievance procedure. Who makes decisions regarding challenged materials or complaints?

School Board?______ Individual?______ Committee?______

How is committee selected?__________

Who is on the committee?__________

If parents object to an assignment, will an alternative assignment be provided without penalty?

____

5. PARENTAL INVOLVEMENT

How are parents notified of program?__________

Is parental permission required for elementary school?__________

middle school?__________ for high school?__________

Where are materials available for parental review?__________

What methods are used to involve parents?__________

6. PROGRAM INFORMATION

In what grades and subjects does the program occur?__________

____

Are there written guidelines/protocols for answering questions? ______

What outside agencies, organizations are used?__________

7. PREGNANT STUDENT PROGRAMS

When a student thinks she might be pregnant:

Are referrals made to local agencies for pregnancy tests?__________

For adoption?__________ For abortion?__________

To what agencies or organizations is the student referred?__________

____

MAKE SEVERAL COPIES BEFORE COMPLETING

Does the district have a policy regarding parental notification when a student suspects she is pregnant? ______

What programs exist for pregnant students carrying babies to term? ______

______

8. COUNSELING AND HEALTH SERVICES

To what agencies or organizations do the schools refer students for:

Health services? ______

Counselors? ______

What resource materials does the district use (i.e., booklets, literature, etc.) for counseling and health services? ______

______

Does the school district have a policy regarding notifying parents if a student suspects he/she has a sexually transmitted disease? ______

9. MISCELLANEOUS COURSES

Apart from a program entitled "Sex Education" or "Family Life Education" described in question 1, what related information is covered in other courses?

	anatomy	physiology	reproduction	STDs	values	issues	other
Biology							
Health							
Phys. Ed.							
Science							
Human Development							
Child Development/ Parenting							
Psychology							
Social Studies							
Decision-Making							

Are teachers of English, history, math and other subjects unrelated to human sexuality allowed to discuss human sexuality in their courses? ______

MAKE SEVERAL COPIES BEFORE COMPLETING

APPENDIX

K

Abstinence Programs Elsewhere in Your Region

Name or Organization/School__________

Contact Person__________

Address__________

City__________ State__________ Zip__________

Phone__________

Name of abstinence curriculum__________

Grade level(s) where used__________

Who teaches it?__________

When was it adopted?__________

What led them to adopt the program?__________

What was the situation before they adopted the program?

____

Has the curriculum helped?__________

Who selected the curriculum?__________

How do teachers like the program?__________

How do parents like the program?__________

How do students like the program?__________

Do they have any newspaper clippings regarding the program?__________

If so, will they mail you copies?__________

Can you use their name as a future reference?__________

Miscellaneous notes:__________

____

____

____

____

____

MAKE SEVERAL COPIES BEFORE COMPLETING

APPENDIX

L

Evaluating Your School's Sex Education Program

Name of material:______________________________

Overall theme:______________________ Grades used in:______________________

Type: ______Book ______Booklet ______Flyer ______Film

______Video ______Slide presentation ______Lesson Plan

______Student Workbook

______Other______________________________

3-4 main messages:______________________________

____

____

Subtle messages:______________________________

____

____

Values represented:______________________________

____

____

Positive values:______________________________

____

____

Negative values:______________________________

____

____

Clear right or wrong?______________________ Good role models?______________________

How does it portray parents?______________________________

____

____

MAKE SEVERAL COPIES BEFORE COMPLETING

PROBLEM AREAS:

Is there a mixed message ("don't do this, but if you do...")?____________________

Does it suggest contraceptives for unmarried teenagers?____________________

Does it suggest abortion by portraying parenthood unfavorably?____________________

Is deviant sexual activity presented as acceptable or normal? (Is deviant sex mentioned, but not defined as deviant or unusual?)____________________

Does it refer to partners instead of husband and wife or spouse? ____________________

Does it suggest postponing sex instead of waiting until marriage? ____________________

Does it refer to long-term relationship instead of marriage?____________________

Is the approach non-directive (providing only facts or leaving evaluation to the student) with no clear advocacy of abstinence?____________________

Is the emphasis on feelings?____________________ On pleasure?____________________

Is self-control minimized? ____________________ Is it too graphic?____________________

OTHER COMMENTS:

Produced by:____________________

Well-known actors____________________

Who selected the material?____________________

Who approved?____________________

MAKE SEVERAL COPIES BEFORE COMPLETING FORM

APPENDIX

M

Giving a Talk Before an Audience

Before you give a talk before a school board, civic association, church or other group, pray for God's guidance throughout your preparation and presentation. Study the scriptures listed in Appendix N.

I. FIND OUT ABOUT THE AUDIENCE AND OCCASION

1. Analyze who your audience will be.
   What is the organization?
   What does the group stand for?
   How do group members feel about your views?
   How many people will be in attendance?
2. Find out what your exact time limits will be.
3. Find out the exact time, date, and location of the meeting.
4. Find out what the layout of the meeting will be.
   Stage? Microphone? Auditorium? Small room?
5. Find out if there will be other speakers at the event. If so, who are the speakers? What are their views? In what order will the speakers give their talks?
6. Will other events take place during the meeting?
7. Will there be questions taken from the audience?

II. DETERMINE YOUR SPECIFIC PURPOSE FOR GIVING A TALK

1. Are you planning simply to inform them about the teenage pregnancy problem in your community?
2. Are you trying to explain to them the dangers of existing programs in the schools?
3. Are you trying to get them to adopt an abstinence program in the schools?
4. Are you trying to change them from a pro-contraceptive view to an abstinence view?

Probably, you will have a combination of the above goals, but keep in mind what you are ultimately aiming to achieve.

III. LIST THE MAIN POINTS YOU WANT TO MAKE

1. Limit the number of main points. Pick out no more than four or five points. If you try to include more than this, you'll overload the audience. Look through *Has Sex Education Failed Our Teenagers?* for ideas as to what you want to convey.

2. Arrange the main points you want to make in your talk. Start out with the problem first, then the solution. Even if your primary purpose is to have objectional materials removed from the classroom, you need to offer the constructive alternative of abstinence education.

   If there will be other speakers who will oppose your views, then include points that will refute their views. Example: "No doubt you will hear people say that the schools need to offer contraceptive education for those who are sexually active, but the truth is that contraceptive information in the classroom sends out a mixed message. Let me explain."

IV. FOR EACH MAJOR POINT, SELECT THE BEST SUPPORTING EVIDENCE TO PROVE YOUR POINT

1. Use the information contained in the sex education report.

2. Use some of the information that you gathered when you did your community profile, your state's laws, your school's policies (or the lack of them), the evaluation of your school's sex education program and places where abstinence is being taught elsewhere in your vicinity.

3. For each major point, use the strongest pieces of evidence.

4. Use a **variety** of types of evidence—some statistics, some charts, some examples, some quotations, some explanations, some definitions, etc. Remember, a talk containing nothing but statistics is dull, and so is a talk containing nothing but quotations.

V. BE SURE TO SHOW HOW THE ISSUE DIRECTLY AFFECTS THE AUDIENCE

1. Talk about their children.

2. Talk about their duties as school board members.

3. Talk about disrupted families.

4. Talk about their goals and how your program meets their needs.

   Example: When talking to the school board, talk about their concern to provide the best programs for their students.

   Example: When talking to a church, talk about how the parents want programs that uphold their Christian values.

   Example: When talking to nurses, talk about how they are interested in promoting good health.

VI. ALWAYS SHOW THESE TRAITS:

1. **PROFESSIONALISM:** You should treat your audience professionally, and you should conduct yourself with dignity.
2. **COURTESY:** Obey the rules. Don't be rude.
3. **GRATITUDE FOR SPEAKING:** Express your appreciation for the opportunity to speak.
4. **APPRECIATION FOR THEIR WORK:** Thank the audience for their involvement in the issue.
5. **EMPATHY TO AUDIENCE:** Regardless of how the audience feels about your views, empathize with the struggles that they are facing.

   Example: It is a tough job to be a good parent today.

   Example: The principal faces many difficult decisions on a daily basis.

VII. PREPARE A WRITTEN DRAFT OF YOUR TALK

1. Use an outline format with complete sentences. Use headings for convenience.
2. Try to type it so that it will be easy for you to read.
3. Use one side of the paper only.
4. Cite the sources of your evidence.
5. Prepare a catchy opening. Close the talk with a conclusion calling for action.

VIII. REHEARSE YOUR TALK

1. Practice your talk aloud several times.
2. Time yourself. The first few times you rehearse it, you'll probably run through it too quickly. Make a point to slow down. If you run overtime during rehearsal, then shorten the content of your speech. DO NOT SPEAK RAPIDLY SO THAT YOU CAN COVER A LOT OF MATERIAL. INSTEAD, SHORTEN YOUR TALK.
3. Ask a friend or family member to listen to your talk. After you rehearse, ask for his or her feedback.
4. Do **not** memorize your speech. Instead, become so familiar with your written outline that you will be able to give a "talk" conversationally.
5. As you rehearse, be sure to look up at your audience. Do not appear to be reading.
6. Practice answering the common questions about abstinence education (see section V. B. in *Has Sex Education Failed Our Teenagers?*).

IX. PREPARE HANDOUTS, IF NECESSARY

1. If you are giving a talk before key decision-makers (i.e. school board), give them a photocopy of your written outline.
2. If you want to give people more information than you can possibly cover in your talk, then prepare a handout.
3. Usually it is best to give the handout at the end of your talk so that people will pay attention to your talk instead of the handout. But if you want to ask people to refer to certain charts during your talk, then pass out the handout before your talk. Explain that you will refer to it at particular points in your presentation.
4. Arrange for a friend to distribute the handouts.
5. Do not pass around small items such as photographs during your speech. They are too distracting.

X. PREPARE VISUAL AIDS, IF NECESSARY

1. Visual aids are an effective means of helping the audience to understand technical information such as statistics, to visualize certain data found on bar graphs, and to focus on key points you wish to emphasize.
2. Look through the sex education report and decide whether some of the tables will help support the points you are trying to make.
3. When selecting or making visual aids, make sure that:
   - they are pertinent to your point;
   - they are clear and simple;
   - they are large enough to be seen from the back of the room;
   - any lettering or numbering is large enough to be read;
   - they are attractive, not sloppy.
4. Practice using your visual aids during rehearsal. Make a note on your written outline reminding you when to show your visual aid.
5. Find out how you will need to display your visual aid at the actual location. You might need to arrange for certain equipment.
6. Show the visual aid only at the proper moment during the speech. Discuss the point you are trying to make with the visual aid. Point to appropriate items on the visual aids. When you have made your point, set the visual aid aside so that it won't be distracting to your audience.

XI. DRESS

1. Find out what the level of formality will be at the meeting.
2. It is usually best for men to dress in a suit and tie, and for women to wear the type of clothes they wear to church. Women need to avoid "girlish" styles.

CHECKLIST BEFORE LEAVING TO GIVE YOUR TALK
Make sure you have—

- ☐ your speaking notes (Bring two copies. Ask your friend to hold onto one in case you lose your copy.)
- ☐ visual aids
- ☐ audiovisual equipment
- ☐ handouts
- ☐ dressed properly
- ☐ address and directions for meeting location
- ☐ notepad so that you can take notes during other people's presentations
- ☐ allowed ample time to arrive early
- ☐ arranged for people to pray for you
- ☐ reviewed the verses on speaking (Appendix N)

XII. ARRIVE EARLY

1. Arrive early in order to get a good seat, to set up audiovisual equipment if necessary, and to have a brief prayer.
2. Ask one or two close friends or family members to accompany you. They can give you positive feedback during your talk. Also, they can pray for you as you speak.

XIII. GIVE YOUR TALK AS PLANNED

1. Place your outline on the podium but don't look at it excessively. Instead, look at the audience as much as possible.
2. Stand in an upright position that is comfortable for you. Don't lean on the podium.
3. Use gestures. Otherwise, keep your arms at your side.
4. Feel free to move around some, unless you're speaking with a stationary microphone.
5. Use your natural voice.
6. Speak loudly enough so that the people in the back can hear. Don't wait until you walk up to the microphone to see if the people in the back can hear you. (When you arrive early, ask your friend to go to the back of the room so that you can test out your volume.)

7. If you forget a point or if you make a mistake, pause for a second. Then pick up where you left off. Don't be afraid if you lose your train of thought, if you feel nervous, or if you make mistakes. You might feel tempted to apologize to the audience, but **don't.** They aren't aware of your nervousness or your mistakes unless you point them out.

XIV. HANDLING QUESTIONS

1. Welcome Questions

Whether you are giving a talk, conducting a press conference, or going before the school board, anticipate that you will be asked questions. Unlike a planned message, answering questions requires an impromptu response. Do not be afraid of questions—welcome them because they can give you the opportunity to strengthen your position.

2. Size Up the Situation

When asked a question, quickly evaluate the person asking the question. Is the person favorable or hostile to your views? Is the person seeking additional information, or is the person seeking clarification of something that you said? Is the person raising a common objection such as the myths listed in section V. B. of *Has Sex Education Failed Our Teenagers?* Also, what can you discern about the person's attitude toward the subject? Toward you? Does the person seem adequately informed about the subject? Considering these questions can help you frame your response most effectively for that person.

3. Use Smooth Transitions

As you begin to respond to the questions addressed to you, offer a short transitional statement such as "A very good question...," "I'm glad to hear somebody ask that question...," "That's a question that many people ask...."

4. Respond to Disagreement

If you sense that the person asking the question does not agree with you, then compliment the person for his or her willingness to enter into a dialogue on the subject. Here are a few examples to use before you give your answer: "I think I can see where you're coming from...," "A lot of people start out with that viewpoint until they examine all the evidence...," "Many people ask that question because they have only had the opportunity to read the reports presented from one perspective. Let's see what else there is on the subject . . . ."

5. Respond to Opposing Information

Sometimes a person who opposes your view will toss out a piece of information assuming that it will prove his or her viewpoint and then ask you to respond to it. Usually this technique is intended to leave you speechless. When a person does this, rephrase their point in less emotional terminology. If the person has not cited the source of the information shared, ask for the particular report or group from which they obtained their data. If it is something from Planned Parenthood, then turn the tables in your direction and point out that Planned Parenthood has also given us more information that calls into question whether their proposal should be accepted. For example, if a person says that Planned Parenthood has called for comprehensive sex education in order to reduce the teenage pregnancy rate, then cite some of the studies from the sex education report that show that Planned Parenthood's own studies show the ineffectiveness of their approach.

6. Tips for Handling a Dominating Opponent

As you answer questions, be brief and factual. Don't let a person dominate the questions. If that occurs, then simply say "Let's give other people the opportunity to ask questions." If nobody else asks questions, then close the questioning session. If the heckler persists, invite him or her to come to you personally to discuss these concerns, rather than take time from the whole group.

APPENDIX

N

Useful Verses to Review Before Speaking

SET AN EXAMPLE AS A CHRISTIAN

Don't let anyone look down on you because you are young,
but set an example for the believers in speech,
in life, in love, in faith and in purity.

—1 Timothy 4:12

LET THE HOLY SPIRIT CONTROL YOU

My message and my preaching
were not with wise and persuasive words,
but with a demonstration of the Spirit's power,
so that your faith might not rest on men's wisdom,
but on God's power.

—1 Corinthians 2:4-5

DO NOT FEEL INADEQUATE—RELY ON GOD

Moses said to the Lord, "O Lord, I have never been eloquent, neither in the past nor since you have spoken to your servant.
I am slow of speech and tongue."
The Lord said to him, "Who gave man his mouth?
Who makes him deaf or dumb?
Who gives him sight or makes him blind?
Is it not I, the Lord?
Now go; I will help you speak and will teach you what to say."

—Exodus 4:10-12

YOUR MESSAGE IS VERY IMPORTANT—YOU KNOW WHAT IS TRUE

I may not be a trained speaker,
but I do have knowledge.

—2 Corinthians 11:6

YOU CAN SPEAK BOLDLY BECAUSE OF THE HOPE GOD HAS GIVEN YOU

Therefore, since we have such a hope,
we are very bold.

—2 Corinthians 3:12

DO NOT BE ASHAMED

I am not ashamed of the gospel,
because it is the power of God
for the salvation of everyone who believes:
first for the Jew, then for the Gentile.

—Romans 1:16

BE BEYOND REPROACH

Similarly, encourage the young men to be self-controlled.
In everything set them an example by doing what is good.
In your teaching show integrity, seriousness and soundness of speech
that cannot be condemned, so that those who oppose you may be ashamed
because they have nothing bad to say about us.

—Titus 2:6-8

POWER OF YOUR SPEECH

The tongue has the power of life and death,
and those who love it will eat its fruit.

—Proverbs 18:21

A wise man's heart guides his mouth,
and his lips promote instruction.

—Proverbs 16:23-24

. . . and pleasant words promote instruction.

—Proverbs 16:21

BE GRACIOUS

Let your conversation be always full of grace.

—Colossians 4:6

BE WISE, NOT FOOLISH

The tongue of the wise commends knowledge,
but the mouth of the fool gushes folly.

—Proverbs 15:2

CONTROL YOUR ANGER

Better a patient man than a warrior,
a man who controls his temper than one who takes a city.

—Proverbs 16:32

A fool gives full vent to his anger,
but a wise man keeps himself under control.

—Proverbs 29:11

HANDLING OPPONENTS

Do not answer a fool according to his folly,
or you will be like him yourself.
Answer a fool according to his folly,
or he will be wise in his own eyes.

—Proverbs 26:4-5

A gentle answer turns away wrath,
but a harsh word stirs up anger.

—Proverbs 15:1

Whoever corrects a mocker brings on insult;
whoever rebukes a wicked man incurs abuse.
Do not rebuke a mocker or he will hate you;
rebuke a wise man, and he will love you.
Instruct a wise man, and he will be wiser still;
teach a righteous man and he will add to his learning.

—Proverbs 9:7-9

APPENDIX

0

Outline of a Sample Talk

OPENING

How would you like to reduce the teenage pregnancy rate in our community by 90%? That's what happened in San Marcos, California, when the school system adopted an abstinence education program. Right now, in our city, we have a high teenage pregnancy rate, not to mention a high rate of abortion and sexually transmitted diseases. But we can change that!

I. TEENAGE SEXUALITY PROBLEM IN OUR COMMUNITY

A. Teenage pregnancy rate
B. Abortion rate
C. STD
D. Physical and psychological problems

II. FAILURE OF PREVIOUS EDUCATION ATTEMPTS

A. The failure of community family planning clinics
B. The failure of comprehensive sex education

III. A SOLUTION THAT WORKS—ABSTINENCE EDUCATION

(At this point you might show the video "Abstinence Education Works—Here's How!")

A. What is abstinence education?
B. Evidence that it works
C. Where abstinence education has been adopted elsewhere in our state

IV. WHAT ACTION THE AUDIENCE MUST TAKE

A. Parents can
   1. Tell teachers, principals, nurses, and others that they want abstinence taught in the schools
   2. Call and write the school board members asking them to adopt a policy which requires the teaching of abstinence education
B. School board members can adopt a policy which requires the teaching of abstinence education

CONCLUSION

(Include a strong appeal that will make the audience realize that their involvement is vital.) Our situation is somewhat like the old man who tried to sell his old violin. The auctioneer opened the bidding at $500. But there were no takers. "Do I hear $100?" There was silence. "Do I hear $50?" Still silence. "What about $10?" But absolutely no takers.

Then out from the audience came the old man who was putting his violin up for sale. He quietly picked up the violin and began playing. He played a song that was beautiful and pleasing to the audience. He then set the violin down and returned to his seat. Suddenly, the audience knew the value of the violin.

The violin sold for $5,000!

Abstinence education is like that old violin—some modern thinkers scoff at it. But to those of us who have learned to cherish its worth, we know it is priceless.

APPENDIX

P

Common Arguments and How to Answer Them

THEY SAY	WE SAY
Teenagers are going to be sexually active.	Not all teens will be. We need to expect the best. (See Section IV.D. of *Has Sex Education Failed Our Teenagers? A Research Report.*)
Teens won't accept the abstinence message.	If they won't accept a clear message of the positive values of abstinence, what makes you think they will accept a contraceptive message? But teens do want an abstinence message. (See Section V.B. 4 and 6 of the sex education report.)
They need to know how to protect themselves.	The best protection is abstinence. Are you willing to take responsibility for recommending teens use methods that have a significant failure rate and carry a risk of life-threatening disease such as AIDS? (See Section III of the sex education report.)
Telling teens to abstain is preaching.	Abstinence is the healthiest choice for teens. (See Section V.B.1. of sex education report.)
Telling teens to abstain is imposing your morals.	By saying that premarital abstinence is moral, you are saying that premarital sexual activity is immoral; I agree with you. (See Section V.B.2. of sex education report.)
Teens need to know the facts.	I agree; but facts should be age-appropriate, and facts alone have not helped reduce teen promiscuity, pregnancy or abortion. Giving facts without values is like teaching a teen how to drive without teaching the rules of the road.

THEY SAY	WE SAY
You can't legislate morality.	All laws are based on morality. (See Section V.B.5. of sex education report.)
Teaching premarital abstinence will offend parents who are living with someone to whom they are not married.	If we accept that reasoning, then we cannot teach right or wrong, good or bad, about such things as stealing, drug and alcohol abuse, lying or respect, because someone might be offended. (See Section V.B.7. of sex education report.)
Yes, abstinence is best. But some teens need to know about birth control.	The best birth control is **self-control.** Birth control has no place among unmarried teens. (See Section III of the sex education report.) If you discuss contraception in a class, you are sending a mixed message to teens. (See Section V.D. of sex education report.)

APPENDIX

Q

Complaint Inquiry

SAMPLE LETTER

Dear M____. ____:

Our organization is a group of parents and interested citizens desiring to contribute positive support to our public schools. We desire to serve the community by promoting interaction on a variety of education issues.

The purpose of this letter is to ask for information regarding a concern brought to our attention by a parent. So that we can gain a better understanding of the situation, we would like for you to complete the enclosed inquiry form and return it to us. It would be helpful if you could enclose a copy of policies or guidelines related to this matter.

This inquiry is not intended to be a complaint or a criticism. If the parent decides to pursue the matter, we will make a referral to the appropriate person or office.

We welcome your comments and will appreciate your response.

Sincerely,

(your name)
(title)

INFORMATION REQUEST

Nature of Concern

______Student assignment ______Literature ______Class discussion

______Policy matter ______Student handout ______Film/video/slides

______Textbook ______Class work ______Other

School:____

Class:____

Teacher:____

______Copy of material enclosed.

Description of Concern or Related Information

Please complete the following:

Does ______________________________________ comply with district policies and guidelines? If not, please explain.

____

____

What was the purpose of the activity?_________________________________

____

Is the activity an unusual one?______________________________________

From what source was this activity generated? (Teacher's materials, textbook, workshop, etc.)?

____

____

Is it your opinion that the activity is appropriate?__________________

What action do you recommend that the parent take?____________________

____

What action, if any, will you take?__________________________________

____

What action, if any, does the school district plan to take?___________

____

MAKE SEVERAL COPIES BEFORE COMPLETING

Other information requested:

____

____

____

____

Comments:____

____

____

____

MAKE SEVERAL COPIES BEFORE COMPLETING

APPENDIX

R

Specific Helps For Parents

1. Be informed

Read books by Christian authors dealing with educational and family issues. Listen to informative radio programs. Know what is going on in your community, state, and country.

2. Be organized

Clip and file newspaper articles related to all areas of education. Date articles and underline names with a red pencil.

a. **Keep a notebook.** At the beginning of the school year, enter your children's class schedule, teachers' names, and teachers' consultation period. Jot down the date of all calls and conferences with teachers, counselors, and the principal. Record the person you spoke with, and a brief summary of the conversation.

b. **Keep a copy of all correspondence** (yours and theirs).

c. **Set goals** for conferences, calls, or letters:
   - Identify the purpose: Is it to gather information, to state your purpose, to request action?
   - Plan what you want to say.
   - List possible solutions to a problem. Then evaluate which ones are acceptable and which ones are not.
   - Ask for copies of rules, guidelines, and policies.

3. Take action

a. Begin and end everything with prayer.

b. Use good grammar, be polite, avoid sensationalism, respect authority.

c. Follow the proper procedure or chain of command: Teacher, department head, principal, district staff superintendent, school board (ask for organizational chart).

d. Be ready to back up your position with facts.

e. Express sincere appreciation whenever possible.

f. Address one issue at a time and stick to it. You may have to repeat a question until you get an answer. Don't be afraid of silence. Wait for an answer.

g. Gather information before you draw conclusions. Ask direct questions.

h. Avoid personal attacks and do not become defensive.

i. Don't assume. Make sure you understand by asking questions such as, "Would it be accurate to say that you believe/think/feel . . .?"

j. Be sure to question or verify information, i.e., "Is that a policy?" "May I see that policy?" "Whose decision is that?"

k. If an action is promised, ask "when? how? who?" etc. Conclude a conversation or letter with, "Then I can expect to hear from you on Monday?" or "I'll expect to hear from you by Friday."

4. Be cautious

If your name or your group's name has been in the paper, or you have spoken at a public meeting, be leery of phone calls seeking information. Someone may be trying to obtain material that can be used against you. Ask questions to determine the caller's motives. For example, "How did you learn about our group?" If the answer is another organization, ask who made the referral and how they happened to contact that organization.

GUIDING PRINCIPLES FOR PARENTS

Parents are accountable to God for the education of their children.

School boards should reflect community values.

You cannot be responsible for the whole world, but you can be responsible for doing what you know is right and trusting the results to God.

Opposition helps make you sharper. You'll learn to express your thoughts and beliefs better and develop a stronger case for your position.

Pursue your objective because it is right, even knowing you may lose. Sometimes you lose a battle, but gain ground. If you lose, that may be the impetus needed to open the eyes of the silent and passive majority.

The manner in which you pursue your objective can strengthen your position and weaken the opposing position, whether you win or lose.

The king's heart is in the hand of the Lord;
he directs it like a watercourse wherever he pleases.

—Proverbs 21:1

Conflict is sometimes necessary to bring about positive change.

Reason changes minds; God's Word changes hearts.

Someone's values will be represented in the media—on radio talk shows, in letters to the editor, guest columns, etc.—why not yours?

If not you, who? Jeremiah said he was too young and Moses said he couldn't speak. Paul said, *I can do everything through him who gives me strength.* Philippians 4:13

Kings take pleasure in honest lips;
they value a man who speaks the truth.

—Proverbs 16:13

APPENDIX

S

Sample Petition

WHEREAS, Today's children and teenagers are bombarded with an increasing amount of societal and media pressure to be sexually active; and

WHEREAS, There is a need for cooperation on this very important issue among parents, churches, and schools; and

WHEREAS, ____________________ in ____________________ believe sex education is a parental responsibility that should be supported by the roles that schools may choose to play; and

WHEREAS, There is no values-neutral curricula, the attempt to label material in certain education-related curricula as values-neutral is offensive to the religious convictions of many school children, their families, and teachers; and

WHEREAS, The attempt to use this mislabeled material often encourages and promotes experimental and promiscuous activities;

Therefore, be it RESOLVED, That, we the representatives of ____________________ in ____________________ encourage parents to become involved in the sex education process through:

1) Sensitivity to the sexual development and learning needs of their own children;
2) Involvement in and communication with their local educational process in review and selection of educational materials;
3) Participation in the political process by encouraging our state legislators to mandate the teaching in the public schools of abstinence until marriage, and to reject all forms of legislation that would permit or require teaching the acceptability of the practices of promiscuous and perverse lifestyles.

Be it finally RESOLVED, That ____________________ in ____________________ encourages and urges our school boards, school administrators and all educators to:

1) Adopt curricula that stress traditional family values as the ideal.
2) Adopt curricula that are true, healthy, legal, and constitutional.
3) Adopt a policy to establish a parental review process in advance of program implementation. That process should be open and effectual, providing parents with the option that their children not participate.

4) Adopt curricula that teach sexual abstinence before marriage and fidelity in marriage as the only acceptable lifestyle in terms of public health, as this is the best and only sure way crisis pregnancies and sexually transmitted diseases can be prevented.

5) Refrain from distribution of condoms and other contraceptive materials.

6) Oppose the establishment of school based clinics which provide sexual counseling.

(Based on a resolution passed by the Southern Baptist Convention, 1987.)

APPENDIX

T

Sample Letters to the Editor

IF YOU WANT TO OBJECT TO WHAT IS BEING TAUGHT IN THE SCHOOLS:

Editor:

Recently, I had the opportunity to review (**film, book, program, or whatever**) which is part of (**course, subject, or whatever**) at (**school**). I felt that it was inappropriate because (**state your reason**). I decided to do some research about the subject, and I found out that several studies confirm my views. According to (**cite one or more studies**), sex education courses that teach (**state what was being taught**) are harmful to teenagers. Specifically, that approach to sex education (**state what it does**).

On the other hand, education which promotes sexual abstinence has been shown to (**list some of the positive effects of abstinence education**).

I encourage parents to let school teachers, nurses, and principals know that you want them to adopt programs that promote adolescent abstinence.

Sincerely,
(**your name**)

IF THERE ARE NO PROBLEMS WITH THE PROGRAMS AT YOUR SCHOOL, BUT YOU WANT THEM TO ADOPT ABSTINENCE EDUCATION:

Editor:

Did you know that the teen pregnancy rate in San Marcos, California, dropped by 90% after the schools adopted a program that promotes adolescent abstinence?

Many school districts in our state are following that pattern, also—including (**cities**).

I urge people to contact their school teachers, nurses, and principals and encourage them to adopt this type of program in our schools.

Sincerely,
(**your name**)

TO REFUTE WHAT WAS REPORTED IN THE MEDIA:

Editor:

On (**date**), (**name of newspaper or TV station**) reported (**what they reported**). That view is very popular, but reputable studies disprove that belief. According to (**list a study**), the truth is that (**a brief summary of what the study showed**). This conclusion is further substantiated by (**another study**), which showed that (**a brief summary of what the study showed**).

In view of this information, it is important for the public to (**reject a particular program? adopt abstinence education?**).
Sincerely,

(your name)

LETTER TO THE EDITOR USED IN A SUCCESSFUL SCHOOL BOARD CAMPAIGN

Editor:

In 1983, the National Commission on Excellence in Education issued a report, "A Nation at Risk," stating that the "educational foundations of our society are presently being eroded by a rising tide of mediocrity that threatens our very future as a nation and a people." It went on to say, "if an unfriendly foreign power had attempted to impose on America the mediocre educational performance that exists today, we might well have viewed it as an act of war."

By 1988, Education Secretary William Bennett said that there had been little progress since then and warned that we are still at risk. Despite the reforms, increased spending, special programs, legislation, etc., many studies and reports confirm what Bennett says.

"A Nation at Risk" tells parents, "You have the right to demand for your children the best our schools and colleges can provide. Your vigilance and your refusal to be satisfied with less than the best are the imperative first step."

There are some answers. Parents are responsible for the education of their children. We must assume more of that responsibility by involving ourselves at every level. We must fight to restore local control. We must return to proven educational methods. We must return to the original purpose of public schools—the education of our children; and we must eliminate unsuccessful programs attempting to treat all the social ills of our society. We must emphasize rigorous academic content over processes and teaching methods. When academic courses deal with value-oriented subjects, we must uphold the highest moral values and expectations—such as the "say no" approach to drugs and to sex before marriage. We must insist on a disciplined atmosphere in the classroom by supporting teachers. We must treat students with respect and expect the best of them.

We must elect legislators and state and local school board members who represent the above views. We can begin by electing (__________**name**__________) and (__________**name**__________) to the (__________**name**__________) School District on (____**date**____).
Sincerely,

(your name)

SAMPLE LETTER ENDORSING A NEW POLICY

Editor:

The (__________name____________) school board and administrators have acted courageously in adopting a strong abstinence-based sex education policy. To fly in the face of the "safe sex" and "they're going to do it anyway" mentality takes boldness and integrity.

To the detractors of this policy, I say: Of course young people will "do it anyway" when you expect them to and tell them how to do it "safely." Explain to a 12-year-old how to drive a car, but don't tell him he's too young to drive and don't explain the consequences of unsafe driving. Omit explaining the rules of the road. Assume he will not be able to control his urge to drive and leave the keys laying around "just in case." Make derogatory comments about those who might inflict their standards of morality, i.e. law enforcement officers. Adopt the idea that most kids his age are doing it. Advise him it would be better to wait until he's older, but give the kid a "fuzz buster." Then expect society to pay for the damages when he succumbs to his urge and takes the car out for a little fun.

The (________name__________) school board's action sends a clear and positive message. The teachers and administrators who will implement this new policy deserve the active support of the total community.

Sincerely,

(your name)

APPENDIX

U

Sample Press Releases

FOR IMMEDIATE RELEASE

CONTACT: (Name of Contact Person)
(Phone number for contact person)

On (**date**), (**name of your organization**) passed a resolution calling for traditional family values to be stressed in public schools in the area of sex education. The resolution is directed toward school boards and administrators. It urges the adoption of policies and curricula which uphold abstinence from sexual activity before marriage and fidelity in marriage as the only acceptable lifestyle in terms of public health, and the only sure way to avoid crisis pregnancies and sexually transmitted diseases.

(**Name**), (**title**) of (**organization**), believes that it is important for schools to uphold a high standard and to expect teenagers to exercise self-control. (**She/He**) said, "For too long schools have attempted to take a value-neutral position in sex education. It is not enough to just provide facts; a standard must be upheld."

A key element in the resolution calls for school districts to provide for a parental review process of programs and materials, and informed parental consent before students participate in sex education programs. The resolution also urges school districts to oppose school based health clinics because these clinics eventually distribute contraceptives to teenagers without parental notification or consent.

(**Name of your organization**) urges other local organizations and churches to present the resolution to their membership for consideration. A copy of the resolution can be obtained by calling (**organization**) at (**phone number**).

FOR IMMEDIATE RELEASE

CONTACT: (Name of Contact Person)
(Phone number for contact person)

(**Organization**) announces its strong support of the proposed sex education policy being considered by the (**name**) school district. This policy would require that public schools uphold the standard of premarital abstinence and fidelity in marriage when they teach sex education. "This is the only responsible approach," states (**name**), (**title**) of (**organization**).

Public schools have the opportunity and responsibility when they teach sex education to uphold a high moral and health standard. The past twenty years of sex education have experimented with providing facts from a so-called "value-free" perspective. This approach has not worked. Providing contraceptive information and services has only worsened the teen pregnancy problem and given a "stamp of approval" to teen promiscuity. Such procedures should be immediately replaced by one of the many successful "abstinence education" curricula which are available for public schools.

Our teenagers need to know the truth that saving sex for marriage is the healthiest choice they can make. This knowledge will free them from the fearful and tragic physical and emotional consequences of unwanted crisis pregnancies and sexually transmitted diseases.

(**Organization**) believes that the proposed new policy demonstrates a concern for excellence and is in the best interest of all public school students. "We call on all concerned parents to encourage our school board members to adopt this policy," said (**name**), (**title**).

(**Organization**) in (**City/County**) is a local chapter of the national (**organization**).

APPENDIX

V

Sample School Board Candidate Screening Forms

(For Nominating Committee)

NOTE: These samples include references to other issues which may be of concern in a local school district.

CANDIDATE SCREENING SURVEY

On a separate sheet of paper, please address the items listed below. Be as clear and concise as possible, while providing adequate information.

1. What is your background and/or experience that you feel would help your candidacy, and be beneficial if elected?
2. Why do you want to be a board member?
3. What clubs, associations and organizations do you currently belong to or have belonged to in the last 5 years?
4. What positions have you held in the community?
5. What current and previous jobs have you held?
6. Describe the following in relationship to being a board member: your temperament, your willingness to study the issues, your willingness to stand alone if you believe you are right.
7. What is your current church affiliation?
8. List three references who know you well.
9. What changes would you work to implement as a board member?
10. Please give your position on the following issues:

Sex Education	Home Schooling
Values Clarification	School-Based Health Clinics
Creation/Evolution	Phonics method of reading

SAMPLE LETTER TO SCHOOL BOARD CANDIDATE

Dear Candidate,

Congratulations on your decision to run for school trustee!

In order to encourage community awareness of candidates and their position on the issues, we are conducting a survey. The results of the survey will be made available to groups, organizations, and news media in the community.

Please carefully note the following instructions:

1. Answer all questions "Yes," "No," or "Undecided." If you choose not to answer a question, a "No Response" answer will be reflected.
2. Please return the completed questionnaire in the next day's mail.
3. Although you are welcome to include comments, they may not be included in the survey report due to space limitations.
4. If your completed survey is not returned by our printing deadline, we will indicate that you did not respond to our survey.

Note: Some questions may be eliminated in the final survey report.

Your response will be appreciated. If you have questions about this survey or its use, please call me.
Sincerely,

(your name)

SAMPLE CANDIDATE SURVEY

1. Should the phonics method be the primary method of teaching reading?
   ________Yes ________No ________Undecided
2. Should the "sight" or "look-say" method be the primary method of teaching reading?
   ________Yes ________No ________Undecided
3. Are you in favor of values clarification?
   ________Yes ________No ________Undecided
4. Are you in favor of the right of parents to homeschool their children?
   ________Yes ________No ________Undecided
5. Are you in favor of a parents' advisory council (separate from the P.T.A.) for the purpose of parental participation in selection of textbooks, programs, and materials?
   ________Yes ________No ________Undecided
6. Are you in favor of the "say 'no' to sex before marriage" approach to sex education?
   ________Yes ________No ________Undecided
7. Should contraceptive instruction and/or counseling be provided by teachers, school nurses, counselors or other school staff?
   ________Yes ________No ________Undecided
8. Are you in favor of school-based (medical) clinics?
   ________Yes ________No ________Undecided
9. Are you in favor of the right of a woman to have an abortion?
   ________Yes ________No ________Undecided

10. Do you believe that our educational materials should uphold the sanctity of life, including that of the unborn?
________Yes ________No ________Undecided

11. Are you in favor of regularly scheduled guidance or counseling classes for elementary students?
________Yes ________No ________Undecided

12. Were you in favor of the last two years' school tax increases in your district? (Answer should reflect your vote if you are an incumbent)
________Yes ________No ________Undecided

13. If elected, will you initiate efforts to establish policies that reflect your views expressed in the above areas?
________Yes ________No ________Undecided

14. Will you vote against issues and policies that contradict the views you expressed above?
________Yes ________No ________Undecided

CANDIDATE NAME____
(Please print)

CANDIDATE POSITION____________________________________

ADDRESS____

PHONE NUMBER____

SCHOOL DISTRICT_______________________________________

____
(Candidate Signature)

APPENDIX

W

Publishers of Abstinence Education Materials

The following organizations or publishers are producers of abstinence resources for the classroom. These groups are also listed in the appendices of the *Sex Education Report* next to the respective titles of the particular resource. In order to keep up with new forthcoming resources, write to the organizations or publishers, asking to receive their current catalogs and to be placed on their newsletter or mailing list.

*Indicates that the organization/publisher has a Christian perspective, but some of their materials are for public schools. This list does not contain all Christian publishers of books for parents and teens; refer to Appendices CC through GG at the end of this handbook for some helpful listings.

American Life League*
Box 1350
Stafford, VA 22554
(703) 659-4171

Character Curriculum, Inc.
112 E. Church St.
Cuero, TX 77954
(800) 544-0760

Concordia Publishing House*
3558 S. Jefferson
St. Louis, MO 63118-3968
(800) 325-3040

Couple to Couple League
Box 11084
Cincinnati, OH 45211
(513) 661-7612

Focus on the Family*
801 Corporate Center Drive
Pomona, CA 91768
(714) 620-8500

Gospel Films*
Box 455
Muskegon, MI 49443
(800) 253-0413

Human Life Center*
University of Steubenville
Steubenville, OH 43952
(614) 282-9953

Josh McDowell Ministries*
Box 1000
Dallas, TX 75221
(214) 234-0645

Learning About Myself and Others
c/o Anne Nesbit
P.R. #48 Orchard Circle
Pittsfield, MA 01201
(413) 698-2688

Life Cycle Books
P.O. Box 792
Lewiston, NY 14092-0792
(416) 690-5860

National AIDS Prevention Institute
P.O. Box 2500
Culpeper, VA 22701
(703) 825-4040

New Dimension Films
85895 Lorane Highway
Eugene, OR 97405
(503) 484-7125

Project Respect
Committee on the Status of Women
Box 97
Golf, IL 60029
(312) 729-3298

Respect, Inc.
P.O. Box 349
Bradley, IL 60915
(815) 932-8389

Teen-Aid, Inc.
N. 1330 Calispel
Spokane, WA 99201
(509) 466-8679

Vital Signs
P.O. Box 1279
Tryon, NC 28782
(704) 859-5392

Womanity*
1700 Oak Park Blvd., Room C-4
Pleasant Hill, CA 94523
(415) 943-6424

APPENDIX

X

Periodicals That Cover Education Issues

All About Issues
American Life League ▪ Box 490 ▪ Stafford, VA 22554
A monthly magazine that reports news pertaining to pro-life and pro-chastity issues.

The Blumenfeld Education Letter
P.O. Box 45161 ▪ Boise, ID 83711
(208) 322-4440
A monthly letter concerning education issues.

Citizen Magazine
Focus on the Family ▪ Pomona, CA 91799
A monthly magazine devoted to various moral issues confronting the legislature, schools, and other institutions. Gives practical advice for citizens who want to impact their community and country.

Concerned Women for America
370 L'Enfant Promenade SW, Suite 800 ▪ Washington, DC 20024
(800) 458-8797
Membership includes monthly magazine.

Education Newsline
Citizens for Excellence in Education
P.O. Box 3200 ▪ Costa Mesa, CA 92628
Membership includes monthly publication.

The Education Reporter
Eagle Forum ▪ P.O. Box 618 ▪ Alton, IL 62002
(618) 462-5415
An excellent monthly newspaper that is devoted exclusively to educational issues. Covers issues and events throughout the nation such as legislation, policies, education trends, parental concerns, controversial issues, etc.

The Rutherford Report
The Rutherford Institute ▪ P.O. Box 510 ▪ Manassas, VA 22110
Quarterly and monthly publications covering "free speech" and "free exercise" legal issues.

APPENDIX

Y

National Organizations That Have Local Chapters

Citizens for Excellence in Education (CEE)
P.O. Box 3200
Costa Mesa, CA 92628
(714) 546-5931

CEE is a national organization dedicated to returning academic and moral excellence to public schools. Local chapters work to inform, encourage and train parents for action in bringing about position changes in public schools. Parents' chapter manual and training videos available.

Concerned Women for America
370 L'Enfant Promenade SW, Suite 800
Washington, DC 20024
1-800-458-8797

CWA is a national organization with local chapters which promote traditional Christian values, religious freedom, the free enterprise system, and a strong national defense. It also provides legal defense.

Eagle Forum
P.O. Box 618
Alton, IL 62002
(618) 462-5414

Eagle Forum is a national organization of spiritually motivated men and women taking a stand for God, a free country, and God-given values. They are involved in educational, economic, family, moral, and defense issues. Local chapters work to affect policy development and educate the public concerning current issues.

APPENDIX

Z

Glossary of Terms

abstinence—refraining from all sexual activity, which includes intercourse, oral sex, anal sex, mutual masturbation, etc.; the only 100% effective means of preventing pregnancy and the spread of sexually transmitted diseases.

affective—influencing emotions or feelings. Note: Affective learning has become very popular and encourages students to divulge their feelings.

alternative life style—a life style that departs from the traditional style of living based on Judeo-Christian morality, i.e. homosexuality, co-habitation.

birth control—the original meaning simply referred to contraceptives; the meaning has been extended by many to include methods of abortion.

birth rate—a ratio indicating births. It does not include abortions and miscarriages. Sometimes called fertility rate. Not the same as pregnancy rate.

cognitive—knowing. This differs from affective learning which deals with feelings.

commitment—pledge, loyalty, entrust. Note: Most sex education courses do not include life-long commitment as a factor to consider before engaging in sexual intercourse.

compliance—act of getting a person to abide. Note: Many school nurses and counselors attend workshops where they are taught how to get sexually active teenagers to comply with regular usage of contraceptives.

contraceptive education—education that includes information about contraceptives. It usually does not include warnings about harm or failure rates. Usually stresses knowledge about types and how they work. Even if no endorsement is given, a mixed message is conveyed to teens that teen sex is presumed and that they should use contraceptives.

contraceptives—medical or mechanical devices that prevent conception. In the past, the term birth control was used, but birth control has come to include abortion as well. Some forms of contraception can also serve as abortifacients too (i.e. I.U.D.).

curriculum—a planned educational series with clearly stated objectives, lesson plans, and activities designed for classroom use, i.e. *Family Values and Sex Education (F.V.S.E.)* is a curriculum from Focus on the Family.

decision-making—determining choices. Note: Beware of popular approaches to decision-making which simply present the student with an array of choices without pointing students in the direction of the best decision.

department—a major administrative division. Within a school, there is a department of social sciences. A teacher usually serves as department head and interacts with other teachers of that subject.

directive education or counseling—education or counseling which moves the student in a predetermined direction. Most sex education courses do not move students toward abstinence.

director—a middle level administrator in a school district, such as the director of nursing.

essential element—a term that describes basic concepts which are usually mandated for study.

family—the traditional definition refers to a household of people related by blood or law, as well as the relatives of those people. Beware of definitions that simply refer to a household of people.

family life education—a phrase often used instead of "sex education."

family planning—a method of controlling family size and spacing of birth dates of children by use of contraceptives. Sometimes abstinence and abortion are listed as family planning methods.

fertility rate—same as birth rate; not the same as pregnancy rate. Note: "Fertility rate" is sometimes used by health departments and data banks.

fidelity—faithfulness to another; usually refers to marital fidelity.

guideline—a description or outline of how a policy should be carried out.

inclusive—allowing all items to be included. Note: Proponents of comprehensive sex education often criticize abstinence educators of not being inclusive.

latency—the stage of childhood (around 5 yrs. to onset of puberty) when sexual urges and interests remain dormant. Note: Most sex education during this stage can be harmful to children.

mandate—that which is mandatory or required.

monogamy—the state of being married to one person. Note: Some people extend this word to describe non-married relationships.

morality—a system of principles relating to right or wrong behavior. Note: Many sex education courses avoid a discussion of what is right or wrong.

non-directive education or counseling—education or counseling not moving students in a predetermined direction. Note: Most sex education courses are non-directive because students are not told what is a morally or practically right choice.

objective—aim, end of a program. Often stated in the form of a behavior.

outercourse—a medical expression used to describe sexual activity which does not culminate in pregnancy or a sexually transmitted disease. Some groups have incorrectly classified some forms of intercourse as outercourse in order to circumvent state laws upholding the teaching of abstinence.

pregnancy rate—a ratio showing the conceptions that occurred. Note: Not the same as birth rate or fertility rate.

policy—a high-level plan embracing the general goals and acceptable procedures.

postponing sexual involvement—the delaying of the onset of sexual intercourse. Note: Sometimes this is simply translated as getting a 12-year-old child to wait until he or she is 15 years old.

rationale—an explanation of controlling principle; an underlying reason for a program.

responsible sex—to those who adhere to Judeo-Christian values, responsible sex is premarital abstinence and marital fidelity. In value-neutral sex education, responsible sex usually means using contraceptives.

safe sex—The only 100% safe sex is premarital abstinence and marital fidelity. Note: some people have defined it as the use of contraceptives in order to reduce the likelihood of pregnancy or transmission of sexually transmitted diseases. The latter definition is the most widespread.

safer sex—an alternative word to safe sex, since contraceptives are not 100% effective.

school-based clinic (SBC)—or school-based health clinic, clinics that are housed on a school campus. Most SBCs give contraceptive counseling, prescriptions, or actual contraceptives.

school board—the highest governing body in a school district.

sex education—education about one or more topics such as human growth and development, reproduction, contraception, abortion, dating, etc.

sexually transmitted diseases (STDs)—diseases that are spread by sexual activity (vaginal, oral, and anal intercourse).

superintendent—the head of a school district.

trustee—a board member.

value-free—without values.

value-neutral—without mention of right or wrong; often a factual presentation with no context of right and wrong.

values clarification—an approach in which all choices are acceptable; right and wrong is considered relative, not absolute; often the basis for a 5-7 step decision making process.

venereal disease (VD)—a contagious disease that is typically acquired in sexual intercourse. It has been replaced by the more accurate term, sexually transmitted diseases.

APPENDIX

AA

Books to Guide Parents

These books give practical information on Christian principles and action. For resources that deal with helpful facts about sex education, refer to Appendices CC through GG.

Barton, David. *America: To Pray or Not To Pray.* Aledo, TX: Specialty Research Associates, Inc., 1988. A statistical look at areas of decline since prayer was removed from public schools in 1962. Illustrates the impact on student academics, student morality, student mortality, and other problems, when a nation does not honor God as God.

Barton, David. *The Myth of Separation.* Wallbuilder Press, (P.O. Box 397, Aledo, TX, 79008), 1989. This book provides an understanding of the issue of separation of church and state. It will enable parents to refute arguments concerning the teaching of values and morals.

Chastian, Jane. *I'd Speak Out on the Issues If I Only Knew What to Say.* Ventura, CA: Regal Books, 1987. A book that gives helpful tips on how to speak up and act on the issues of school-based clinics, comparable worth, sex education, pay equity, pornography, abortion, and the equal rights amendment.

Echaniz, Judith. *When Schools Teach Sex.* Rochester, NY: Free Congress Research and Education Foundation, 1982. A handbook giving excellent advice on how to evaluate a sex education program and values clarification.

Educational Guidance Institute. *Curriculum Guidelines for Grade Levels.* Educational Guidance Institute, Inc., 927 S. Walter Reed Drive, Suite 4, Arlington, VA 22204, (703) 486-8313. An excellent list of age-appropriate curriculum guidelines for each grade level.

Gabler, Mel and Norma, with James C. Hefley. *What Are They Teaching Our Children?* Wheaton, IL: Victor Books, 1985. A good book to begin to understand the public school system and its many problems, and what Christians can do about them. Chapters on curriculum, textbooks, sex education, evolution and creation, and what parents can do.

Citizens for Excellence in Education. *How to Get Christians Elected to Public Office.* Costa Mesa, CA: Citizens for Excellence in Education.

Leman, Kevin. *Smart Girls Don't and Guys Don't Either: A Survival Guide for Parents of Teens and Pre Teens.* Ventura, CA: Regal Books, 1982. Helps prepare teens to make smart decisions about peer pressure, choosing friends, sex, drugs, dating, etc.

Mast, Coleen. *Implementation Guide.* Bradley, IL: Respect, Inc. A practical guide which assists those people who want to implement the *Sex Respect* curriculum in their schools.

McDowell, Josh. *Why Wait? Action Packet.* Dallas, TX: Josh McDowell Ministries. A useful resource giving some basic facts about the teenage sexuality crisis, how to get your church to adopt the right program, and resources to use for educating parents and teens.

Schlafly, Phyllis. *Child Abuse in the Classroom.* Alton, IL: Pere Marquette, 1984. Contains excerpts from national hearings where parents testified about school practices in violation of their values. A good section on action.

Whitehead, John. *Parents Rights.* Also *The Christian Duty of Political Involvement: Responsibility and Stewardship.* Ft. Lauderdale, FL: Coral Ridge Ministries, 1984. A booklet about stewardship and responsibility of Christians in the role of civil government.

APPENDIX

BB

Audiovisual Resources for Adults on Teenage Sexuality

Abstinence Education Works—Here's How!

Excellent resource for getting key decision-makers to adopt abstinence education. Good video for a promotional packet. A videotape of Mike Long of Project Respect discussing the importance and effectiveness of abstinence education. Available from: Project Respect. Committee on the Status of Women, Box 97, Golf, IL 60029-0097, (312) 729-3298.

A Critical Look at Planned Parenthood

Excellent tool to convince the community not to allow Planned Parenthood to come into the schools. Two 45-minute slide presentations that take a critical look at Planned Parenthood. Available from: Vital Signs, P.O. Box 1279, Tryon, NC 28782, (704) 859-5392.

How to Stop School-Based Sex Clinics

A 52-minute video which features 20 national leaders who oppose school based clinics. Available from: American Life League, Box 1350, Stafford, VA 22554, (703) 659-4171.

Myths of Sex Education

A 45-minute video in which Josh McDowell examines the secular agenda as it relates to sex education, exposing common myths about comprehensive sex instruction. Available from Josh McDowell Ministries, Box 1000, Dallas, TX 75221, (214) 907-1000.

New Perspectives in Education

A video of a full-day workshop by Dr. William Coulsen, former researcher for Carl Rogers and Abraham Maslow. Dr. Coulsen describes the detrimental effects that humanist psychology have had on our educational system. Available through People for Responsible Education, 420 N. Seventh St., Barron, WI 54812.

Project Sex Respect

A videotape in which LeAnna Benn of Teen-Aid and Coleen Mast of Respect, Inc. give overviews of their public school abstinence curricula. Available from: Womanity, 1700 Oak Park Blvd., Room C-4, Pleasant Hill, CA 94523, (415) 943-6424.

Promo Video: Sex Respect

Excellent resource for getting key decision-makers to adopt abstinence education. Coleen Mast talks about the need for abstinence education in the schools. Available from: Respect, Inc., P.O. Box 349, Bradley, IL 60915-0349, (815) 932-8389.

School-Based Health Clinics

A videotape of two talks given at a national conference. In the first part, Stan Weed, Ph.D., discusses his statistical research showing the failure of teen family planning services. In the second part, Helen Blackwell gives practical advice for opposing SCSs. Available from: Concerned Women for America, 370 L'Enfant Promenade SW, Suite 800, Washington, DC 20024, (800) 458-8797.

School Sex Clinics

A 17-minute videotape exposing the danger of school-based clinics. Available from: Womanity, 1700 Oak Park Blvd., Room C-4, Pleasant Hill, CA 94523, (415) 943-6424.

Where Youth Are Today

A videotape of Josh McDowell talking about the teenage sexuality crisis. From a Christian perspective. Available from: Word Inc., P.O. Box 2518, Waco, TX 76702, (817) 772-7650.

Why Wait Preview Tape

Contains interviews with various national leaders who are calling for a morally based abstinence approach to the teenage sexuality crisis. From a Christian perspective. Also available in the 8-part video series *How to Help Your Child Say 'No' to Sexual Pressure.* Available from: Josh McDowell Ministries, Box 1000, Dallas, TX 75221, (214) 234-0645.

APPENDIX

CC

Books for Teens

These books have a Christian perspective.

Choices: Finding God's Way in Dating, Sex, Singleness, and Marriage. By Stacy and Paula Reinhart. Nav Press.

Dating: Picking and Being a Winner. By Barry St. Clair and Bill Jones. Here's Life.

Dr. Dobson Answers Your Questions. By James Dobson. Tyndale.

Evidence for Joy. By Josh McDowell. Word.

Falling Into the Big "L." By Karen Sandvig. Regal Books.

Givers, Takers, and Other Kinds of Lovers. By Josh McDowell. Tyndale.

Guidebook to Dating, Waiting, and Choosing a Mate. By Norman Wright and Marvin Inmon. Harvest House.

Just Like Ice Cream. By Lissa Halls Johnson. Ronald N. Haynes.

Love, Dad. By Josh McDowell. Word.

Love: Making It Last. By Barry St. Clair and Bill Jones. Here's Life.

Passion and Purity. By Elisabeth Elliot. Revell.

Preparing for Adolescence. By James Dobson. Vision House.

Questions Teenagers Ask about Dating and Sex. By Barry Wood. Revell.

The Secret of Loving. By Josh McDowell. Here's Life.

Sex: Desiring the Best. By Barry St. Clair and Bill Jones. Here's Life.

APPENDIX

DD

Tapes for Teens

These tapes have a Christian perspective.

Biblical Sexuality. Focus on the Family, Pomona, CA 91799, (714) 620-8500.

How to Say No: The More Positive Answer. Josh McDowell Ministries, Box 1000, Dallas, TX 75221, (214) 907-1000.

Maximum Dating. Josh McDowell Ministries (see above).

Maximum Love. Josh McDowell Ministries (see above).

Message to Teens about Sex. Focus on the Family (see above).

Preparing for Adolescence. Focus on the Family (see above).

Preparing for College. Focus on the Family (see above).

Questions Teens Ask. Focus on the Family (see above).

Sexuality and Singles. Focus on the Family (see above).

Sexuality: Letters From Teens. Focus on the Family (see above).

Smart Girls Don't. Focus on the Family (see above).

Straight Talk to Teens about Sex. Focus on the Family (see above)

Strengthening the Marital Bond. Plus a fact sheet on the twelve stages of courtship. Focus on the Family (see above).

Teen Sexuality. Three tapes. Focus on the Family (see above).

Understanding Physical and Sexual Development. Focus on the Family (see above).

Understanding Sexuality. Focus on the Family (see above).

Understanding the Real Meaning of Love. Focus on the Family (see above).

APPENDIX

EE

Books to Help Parents Teach Children

Most of these books have a Christian perspective.

All Grown Up and No Place to Go: Teenagers in Crisis. By David Elkind. Addison-Wesley Publishing.

An Answer to Parent-Teen Relationships. By Norman Wright. Harvest House.

Decent Exposure—How to Teach Your Children About Sex. By Connie Marshner. Wolgemuth and Hyatt.

Gift for All Ages. By Clifford and Joyce Penner. Word.

How to Help Your Child Say No to Sexual Pressure. By Josh McDowell. Word.

How to Teach Your Child About Sex. By Grace Ketterman. Power Books.

The Hurried Child: Growing Up Too Fast Too Soon. By David Elkind. Addison-Wesley Publishing.

Miseducation: Preschoolers at Risk. By David Elkind. Alfred A. Knopf Publisher.

Sex Roles in the Christian Family. By Peter Blitchington. Tyndale House Publishers.

Smart Kids, Stupid Choices. By Kevin Leman. Regal Books.

Talking It Over. By Josh McDowell. Josh McDowell Ministries.

Teens Speak Out. By Josh McDowell. Here's Life.

Why Wait? What You Should Know About the Teenage Sexuality Crisis. By Josh McDowell. Here's Life.

APPENDIX

FF

Tapes to Help Parents Teach Children

These tapes have a Christian perspective.

Developing Your Child's Character. Focus on the Family, Pomona, CA 91799, (714) 620-8500.

Helping Your Kids Say No. Focus on the Family (see above).

How to Teach Your Child About Sex (side 1) and **Sex Education at Home** (side 2). Focus on the Family (see above).

Responsible Sex Education. Focus on the Family (see above).

Teen Sex—A Dangerous Viewpoint. Focus on the Family (see above).

Violence and Teen Sexuality. Focus on the Family (see above).

Where Our Youth Are Today. Focus on the Family (see above).

APPENDIX

GG

Pamphlets to Help Parents Teach Children

These pamphlets are written from a Christian perspective.

Dating and Marriage. InterVarsity Press, P.O. Box 7895, Madison, WI 53707, (608) 836-9765.

Facts of Life: Teaching Your Children About Sex. Focus on the Family, Pomona, CA 91799, (714) 620-8500.

Open Letter to Parents on Teen Sexuality (fact sheet) Focus on the Family (see above).

Preparing for Adolescence. Focus on the Family (see above).

Values in the Home. Focus on the Family (see above).